before the last date shown below.

Oral Medicine

Commissioning Editor: Michael Parkinson

Development Editor: Hannah Kenner

Project Manager: Caroline Horton/Frances Affleck

Design Direction: Stewart Larking

Illustrator: David Gardiner

Oral Medicine

Sergio Gandolfo MD DDS
Professor
Head of the Oral Medicine Section
Department of Biomedical Sciences and Human Oncology
School of Medicine and Surgery
University of Turin, Italy

Crispian Scully CBE MD PhD MDS MRCS FDSRCS FDSRCPS FFDRCSI
FDSRCSE FRCPath FMedSci DSc
Dean, Director of Studies and Research
Eastman Dental Institute University College
University of London, UK

Marco Carrozzo MD DDS
Researcher
Oral Medicine Section
Department of Biomedical Sciences and Human Oncology
School of Medicine and Surgery
University of Turin, Italy

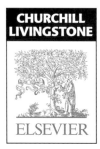

CHURCHILL LIVINGSTONE

ELSEVIER

Edinburgh   London   New York   Oxford   Philadelphia   St Louis   Sydney   Toronto 2006

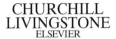

CHURCHILL
LIVINGSTONE
ELSEVIER

English-language edition © 2006, Elsevier Limited. English-language rights reserved.

The rights of Sergio Gandolfo, Crispian Scully and Marco Carrozzo to be identified as authors of this work has been asserted by them in accordance with the Copyright, Designs and Patents Act 1988

ISBN 10: 0443100373
ISBN 13: 2978-0-443-10037-6

This edition 2006
Italian edition 2002, published by Unione Tipografico-Editrice Torinse

British Library Cataloguing in Publication Data
A catalogue record for this book is available from the British Library

Library of Congress Cataloging in Publication Data
A catalog record for this book is available from the Library of Congress

Note
Knowledge and best practice in this field are constantly changing. As new research and experience broaden our knowledge, changes in practice, treatment and drug therapy may become necessary or appropriate. Readers are advised to check the most current information provided (i) on procedures featured or (ii) by the manufacturer of each product to be administered, to verify the recommended dose or formula, the method and duration of administration, and contraindications. It is the responsibility of the practitioner, relying on their own experience and knowledge of the patient, to make diagnoses, to determine dosages and the best treatment for each individual patient, and to take all appropriate safety precautions. To the fullest extent of the law, neither the Publisher nor the Authors assumes any liability for any injury and/or damage to persons or property arising out or related to any use of the material contained in this book.

The Publisher

Contents

Part 3: **Therapy** 143

Chapter 5:
Guide to the main drugs used in the treatment of oral mucosal diseases 145

Chapter 6:
Main drug side effects of oral and perioral localisation 153

Foreword

This text, *Oral Medicine*, written by world renowned experts with a wide clinical experience and a thorough scientific background, is directed on both the dental and medical profession, and rightly so. Oral Medicine is in fact the bridge between medicine and dentistry, if these disciplines should be separated at all.

Oral Medicine combines the features of a classic textbook with a well-illustrated atlas. The authors have structured the book in a rather unique way. Apart from the traditional description of the various diseases and conditions that may be encountered in the oral and perioral tissues, practical guidelines in the form of flowcharts are provided in order to arrive at the most likely diagnosis. Another useful part of this book is the chapter on differential diagnosis by site, in which, based on the clinical appearance, e.g. ulceration, the most common or most likely lesions can be identified. The chapter on drugs that are used in the treatment of oral mucosal diseases and also the chapter on the main side-effect of such drugs are just other examples of the clinical usefulness of this atlas. This also applies to the chapter on how to perform a biopsy of oral lesions.

All together, the authors have accomplished an excellent manual that both provides all necessary information about the various diseases and, at the same time, helps the reader to apply this knowledge in his daily practice. Furthermore, suggestions have been made for various levels of expertise that are required for handling a patient with an oral or perioral lesion, such as a patient with a disease that may be monitored by a general physician or a non-specialised dentist, or a patient with a disease that requires management in a specialist referral centre.

The text is well-written and supported with excellent illustrations and a selected number of references. I can wholeheartedly recommend its use in the daily practice of dentists and physicians and also in the training programmes of undergraduate and graduate students either in the medical or the dental profession.

Isaäc van der Waal
Amsterdam, The Netherlands
2006

Preface

This book is aimed at those training in the field of oral medicine, the discipline to which we have dedicated our teaching, practicing and research activity of many years. It provides different levels of reading that should be useful to dental students, dentists, general practitioners, and specialists from related fields.

Students preparing for university exams need a well-organised text that can help them memorise the notions that are considered fundamental by the scientific community. In order to attain that goal we have adopted the formula of an atlas-type text that contains a comprehensive summary of all the basic information on each disease: clinical aspects, frequency, aetiology, diagnosis and therapy.

Dentists are often the first health professionals to see patients with oral cavity diseases, and have the responsibility of identifying visually and assessing whether they can treat each case or whether they should refer it. They will find everything necessary to resolve this issue easily: diagnostic flowcharts that allow the identification of the most probable diagnosis; basic although comprehensive information about the main diseases that afflict the oral cavity; a colour-coding scheme that indicates the seriousness of each disease; a comprehensive section on drugs and their use in oral medicine; and an accurate description of how to execute different types of biopsy.

General practitioners do not have in their curriculum the same specific training in oral medicine. Despite that, patients suffering from oral conditions often seek the GP's help in the first instance and therefore we are certain that practitioners would be interested in updating their knowledge in this area. We have tried to provide them with a simple text, quick and easy to refer

to, although rigorous and scientifically up to date. We are sure that they will find it very useful, whether it is the diagnostic flowcharts, which, based on the visual appearance of the lesions, easily lead the non-expert eye to the most probable diagnosis, or the sections on the therapy side of our discipline.

Specialists from related fields (dermatologists, maxillofacial surgeons, otorhinolaryngologists), who know oral medicine is very close to their own discipline, will find the overview of this text useful, especially the sections on differential diagnosis and, given that they often see patients who suffer from these diseases, we have included the diagnostic and therapeutic algorithms as a result of an updated revision and summary of the literature.

Furthermore, we expect readers to find the illustrations, specially selected by the authors, particularly useful and we believe they constitute one of the merits of the book.

An illustrated atlas always requires certain efforts on the part of publishers. We acknowledge the work of UTET (the publishers of the original Italian edition) in creating a graphic look for our ideas and we also give thanks to Dr Monica Pentenero and Dr Paolo Giacomo Arduino for invaluable help with the layout of the text. Finally, we thank Martin Dunitz publishers and Stephen Flint, Stephen Porter and Kursheed Moss for all the iconographic material at our disposal from *Atlas of Oral and Maxillofacial Diseases*.

SERGIO GANDOLFO

CRISPIAN SCULLY CBE

MARCO CARROZZO

How to use this book

DIAGNOSTIC FLOWCHARTS

The Diagnostic Flowcharts in Part One follow these principles:

- The basis for diagnosis is the set of *clinical features* and not the disease.

- *Clinical features* are divided into the following six types, which are easily identifiable by the non-expert thanks to the photographs within:

  White or white and red spots and plaques

  Red lesions

  Erosions

  Ulcers

  Blisters and vesicles

  Papillary-verrucous lesions.

With the help of the photographs you can identify which *clinical feature* shows the relevant lesion.

- The flowchart should then be followed according to the arrows, and the questions answered in succession. This leads to the identification of the disease whose name is written in the yellow box; thus reaching *the most likely diagnosis.*

- Finally the disease in question can be found in the Pathology section, Part Two. Each case must then be assessed by comparing the description with the photographs. It must be remembered, however, that a *conclusive diagnosis* is only reached once certain criteria have been met.

The diagnosis protocols and the diagnostic procedures required for a *conclusive diagnosis* could be either simple or complex, in the latter case it must be decided whether the patient should be sent to a specialist referral centre.

In order to assist the readers evaluate the complexity of any specific disease, a **Colour-coding Scheme** has been introduced.

COLOUR-CODING SCHEME

The difficulties for diagnosis and treatment of each disease listed in the Pathology section of Part Two, have been classified according to the following colour-coding scheme:

Green
Patients with a disease that may be monitored by a general physician or a non-specialised odontologist.

Yellow
Patients with a disease that may be monitored by a general physician or a non-specialised odontologist working in conjunction with a specialist unit.

Red
Patients with a disease that should be sent to a specialist referral centre.

Part One

Diagnosis

Chapter One

Differential diagnosis by site

Gingiva

Redness

- Plaque-induced gingivitis
- Trauma
- Odontogenic infections
- Desquamative gingivitis
  - lichen planus
  - pemphigoid
  - pemphigus
- Granulomatous disorders
  - Crohn's disease and other related conditions
  - orofacial granulomatosis
  - sarcoidosis
- Medication
  - plasma cell gingivitis
- Erythroplakia
- Kaposi's sarcoma

Bleeding

- Periodontal disease
- Haemorrhagic disease
- Leukaemia
- Medication

Swelling

- Gingival fibromatosis
- Leukaemia
- Medication
  - phenytoin
  - ciclosporin
  - calcium channel blockers
- Vitamin C deficiency
- Epulides
  - pregnancy epulis
  - fibrous epulis
  - giant cell epulis (could be due to hyperparathyroidism)
- Tumours
- Granulomatous disorders
  - Crohn's disease and related disorders
  - sarcoidosis
  - orofacial granulomatosis

Ulceration

- Necrotising gingivitis

Lips

Angular stomatitis

- Local infections
  - candidosis
  - staphylococcal, streptococcal or mixed staphylococcal-streptococcal infections
- Haematinic deficiencies
  - vitamin B group
  - iron
  - folate
- Immunodeficiency
  - Crohn's disease
  - HIV related infections
  - diabetes

Bleeding

- Trauma
- Cracked lips
- Erythema multiforme
- Angiomas and telangiectasias

Blistering or vesicles

- Herpes labialis
- Burns
- Mucoceles
- Impetigo
- Allergic cheilitis

Peeling and crusting

- Dehydration
- Exposure to the wind
- Fever
- Cheilitis
- Erythema multiforme
- Psychogenic causes
- Medication

Swelling

- Oedema
  - trauma
  - infection (also odontogenic)
  - insect bite
- Angioedema
- Granulomatous disorders
  - Crohn's disease and orofacial granulomatosis
  - sarcoidosis
- Mucoceles
- Tumours
- Abscesses

Ulceration

- Contagious
  - herpes labialis
  - syphilis
  - leishmaniasis
  - deep mycoses
- Tumours

- squamous cell carcinoma
- basal cell carcinoma
- keratoacanthoma
- Burns
- Trauma

Palate

Swelling

- Dental causes
  - unerupted teeth
  - odontogenic cysts
  - abscesses
- Torus palatinus
- Tumours
  - fibrous lumps
  - papillomas
  - squamous cell carcinoma
  - antral carcinoma
  - salivary tumours
  - Kaposi's sarcoma
  - lymphomas
  - other tumours
- Fibro-osseous lesions
  - fibrous dysplasia
  - Paget's disease

Redness

- Candidosis
- Mucositis
- Erythroplasia
- Kaposi's sarcoma
- Pemphigus

Blistering

- Burns
- Pemphigoid
- Localised oral purpura (angina bullosa haemorragica)
- Mucocele
- Pemphigus

Ulceration

- Tumours
  - squamous cell carcinoma
  - salivary tumours
- Necrotising sialometaplasia

Tongue

Swelling

- Congenital
  - lingual thyroid

- haemangioma
- lymphangioma
- median rhomboid glossitis
- foliate papillitis
- Abscesses
- Oedema
  - inflammatory
  - angioedema
- Haematoma
- Foreign body
- Cysts
- Tumours
  - fibrous lumps
  - papilloma
  - squamous cell carcinoma
  - granular cell tumour (myoblastoma)
  - Kaposi's sarcoma

Macroglossia

- Relative macroglossia
  - congenital
    Down's syndrome
    cretinism
    Beckwith's syndrome
  - acquired
  - Ludwig's angina
    angioedema
- True macroglossia
  - congenital
    vascular:
        lymphangioma
        haemangioma
    cysts:
        dermoid cyst
  - acquired
    trauma
    infection
    angioedema
    amyloidosis
    acromegaly
    tumours

Ulceration

- Infectious causes
  - syphilis
  - tuberculosis
  - mycoses
  - herpesvirus infections
- Tumours
  - squamous cell carcinoma
- Trauma
- Aphthous stomatitis
- Drugs

Floor of Mouth

Swelling

- Fibrous hyperplasia
- Odontogenic causes
  - abscesses
- Tumours
  - soft tissue tumours
  - squamous cell carcinoma
  - salivary tumours
- Cysts
  - mucoceles
  - retention cysts

Redness

- Candidosis
- Mucositis
- Erythroplakia

Ulceration

- Tumours
  - squamous cell carcinoma
  - salivary tumours
- Chemical burns
- Aphthous stomatitis
- Drugs

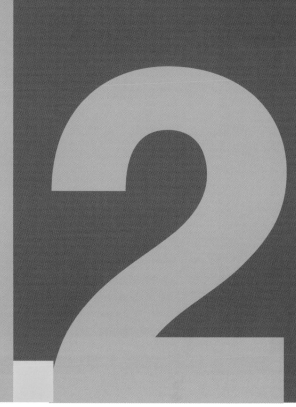

Chapter Two

Differential diagnosis by signs and symptoms

Halitosis

- Oral disease
  - sepsis, poor oral hygiene
  - tumours
  - xerostomia
- Volatile foodstuffs
- Drugs
- Tobacco
- Respiratory tract disease
  - infections
  - foreign bodies
  - tumours
- Metabolic disease
  - liver failure
  - renal failure
  - diabetic ketoacidosis
  - trimethylaminuria
- Psychogenic

Facial Swelling

- Inflammation and infection
- Trauma
- Post-operative emphysema
- Insect bites
- Angioedema
- Endocrine/metabolic causes (corticosteroids)
- Cysts
- Neoplasms
- Haemangioma-lymphangioma
- Foreign bodies
- Granulomatous disorders
  - Crohn's disease
  - sarcoidosis
  - Melkersson–Rosenthal syndrome and granulomatous cheilitis
  - orofacial granulomatosis

Swelling of the Salivary Glands

- Inflammatory
  - mumps
  - HIV infection
  - HCV infection
  - Sjögren's syndrome
  - sarcoidosis
- Obstruction
  - calculi
  - neoplasms
- Tumours
- Sialoadenitis
- Sialosis
- Drugs
- Other

Dry Mouth (Xerostomia)

- Drugs
- Dehydration
- Psychogenic causes
- Salivary gland disease
- Irradiation

Burning Mouth Syndrome

- Deficiency of
  - vitamin B_{12}
  - folic acid
  - iron
  - vitamin B complex
  - other group B vitamins
- Infections (candidosis)
- Erythema migrans (geographic tongue)
- Diabetes mellitus
- Xerostomia
- Psychogenic (somatoform disorder)
- Drugs (e.g. ACE inhibitors)

Pain

- Localised causes
  - odontogenic
  - sinusitis
- Vascular causes
  - migraine
  - giant cell arteritis
- Neurogenic
  - trigeminal neuralgia
  - malignant tumours of the trigeminal nerve
- Herpes zoster (including post-herpetic neuralgia)
- Psychogenic pain
  - atypical facial pain
- Referred pain
  - angina
  - nasopharyngeal, ocular and aural disease
  - chest disease (rare)

Facial Palsy

- Neurological
  - upper motor neurone lesion: cerebrovascular accident
  - lower motor neurone lesion: e.g. Bell's palsy, Lyme disease, HIV, other viral neuropathies
- Middle ear disease

- Parotid lesion
- Trauma to facial nerve branch

Pigmentation

- Racial
- Food/drugs
  - chlorhexidine
  - minocycline
  - zidovudine
- Endocrinological
  - pregnancy
  - Addison's disease
- Others
  - amalgam tattoo
  - lentigines
  - melanoma
  - naevi
  - Peutz–Jegher's syndrome
  - Kaposi's sarcoma

Purpura

- Trauma
- Platelet disorders
- Autoimmune disorders
- Bone marrow disease
  - leukaemia
  - aplastic anaemia
- Infectious diseases
  - infectious mononucleosis
  - rubella
  - HIV/AIDS
- Angina bullosa haemorrhagica
- Amyloidosis

Premature Loss of Teeth

- Immunodeficiency
  - HIV/AIDS
  - cyclic neutropenia
  - Papillon-Lefevre syndrome
- Hypophosphatasia
- Ehlers–Danlos syndrome

Sialorrhoea

- Psychogenic
- Painful oral lesions or foreign bodies
- Drugs
- Cholinergic drugs
- Poor neuromuscular coordination
  - Parkinson's disease
  - facial palsy
  - other weakening diseases

Trismus

- Extra-articular causes
  - infection and inflammation near masticatory muscles
  - temporomandibular joint-dysfunction syndrome (facial arthromyalgia)
  - factured condylar neck
  - fibrosis (scars, irradiation, submucous fibrosis)
  - tetanus toxoid
- Intra-articular causes
  - dislocation
  - intracapsular fracture
  - arthritis
  - ankylosis

Chapter Three

Diagnostic flowcharts

3

White or white and red spots and plaques

These lesions must be differentiated from the *papillary-verrucous* lesions, whose appearance is often white or white and red, is shown in this section and for which there is a different flowchart. If it has been established that the lesions are non-papillary-verrucous then the first question would be:

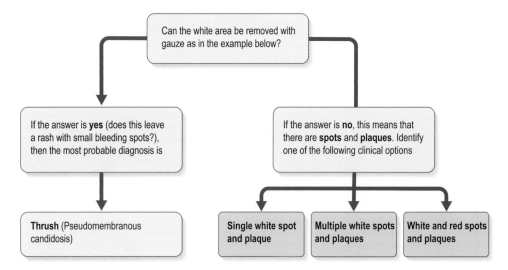

Can the white area be removed with gauze as in the example below?

If the answer is **yes** (does this leave a rash with small bleeding spots?), then the most probable diagnosis is

Thrush (Pseudomembranous candidosis)

If the answer is **no**, this means that there are **spots** and **plaques**. Identify one of the following clinical options

Single white spot and plaque

Multiple white spots and plaques

White and red spots and plaques

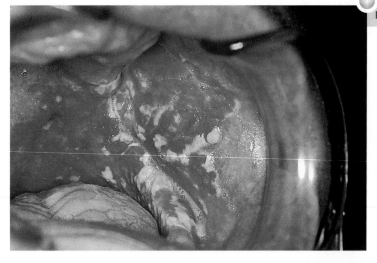

FIGURE 3.1 Clinical aspect of **thrush.**

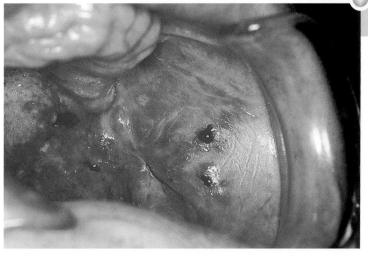

FIGURE 3.2 The same patient after the removal of the **white patches** with gauze.

Single white spot or single white plaque

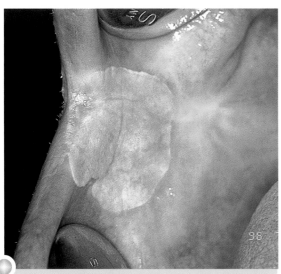

FIGURE 3.3 A **white macule** is a flat lesion simply reflecting a change of the mucosal colour; it may be smooth or finely granular in texture.

Note

A plaque is flatter than a papillary-verrucous lesion ands its surface presents a flat/irregular appearance.

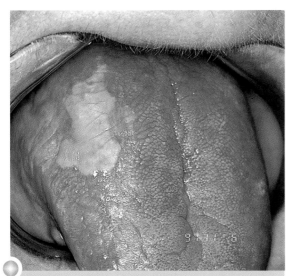

FIGURE 3.4 A white **plaque** is a thickened lesion (thickness ranging from 1 or few millimetres) with a slightly wavy surface, which is usually rough, at times crossed by lines. It can be a few millimetres or many centimetres wide, it varies.

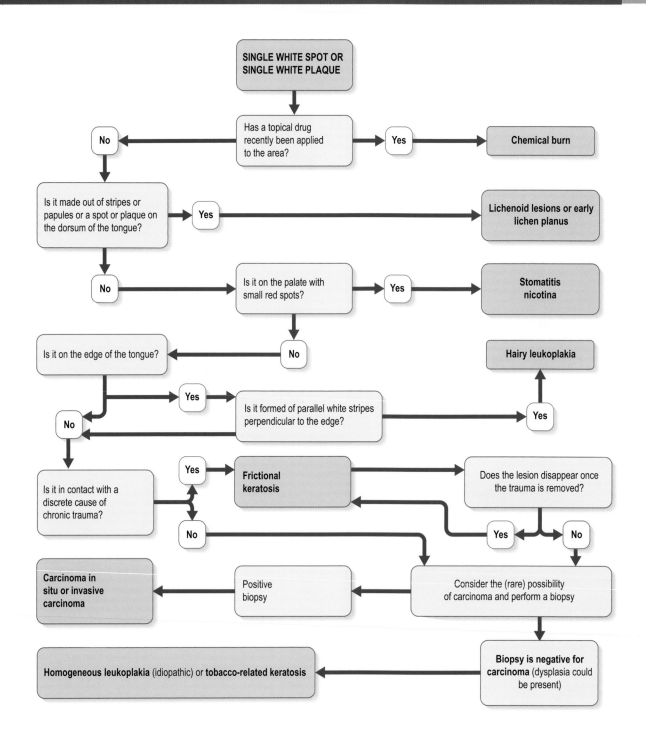

Multiple white spots and multiple white plaques

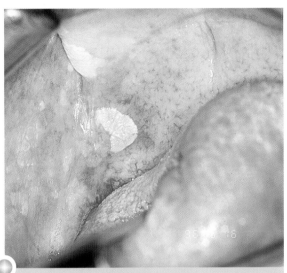

FIGURE 3.5 The **white spots** are similar to those described earlier on but spread over one area or several or the whole mucous membrane.

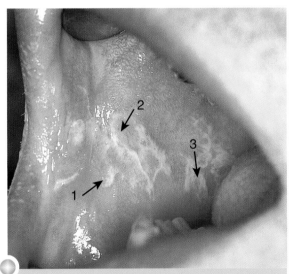

FIGURE 3.6 The **papules (1)** are round white lesions, of small diameter and quite numerous that tend to merge thus creating multiform geometric patterns. Amongst which **white stripes (2)** or the actual **plaques (3)** do stand out clearly.

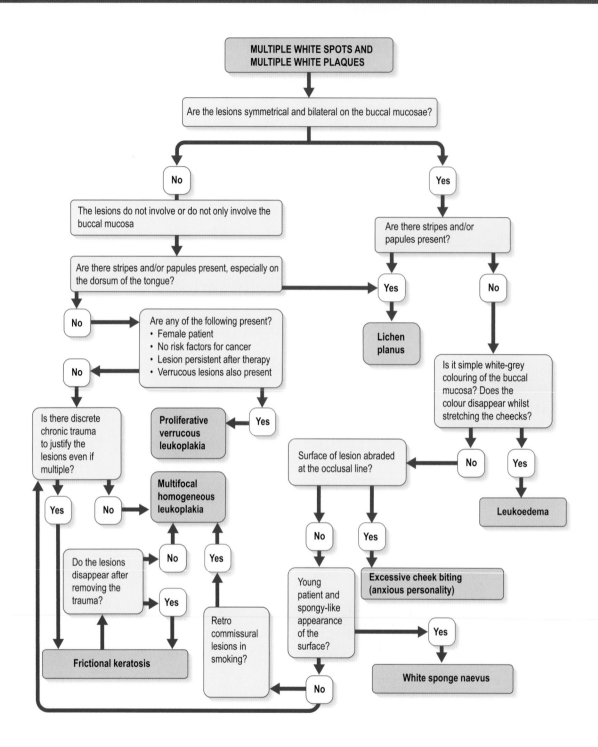

White and red spots and plaques

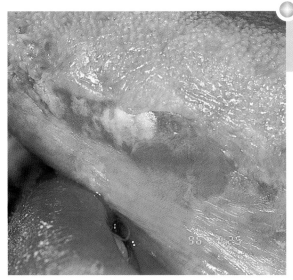

Note

Consider them carefully because this is one of the most frequent appearances of early oral cancer.

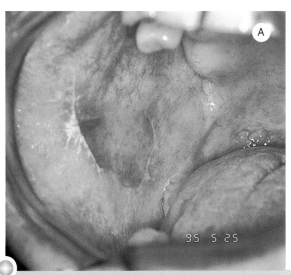
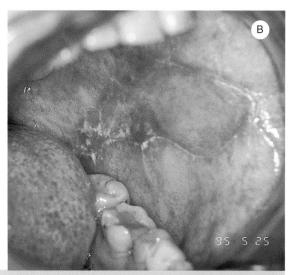

FIGURE 3.8 Another possible aspect is papules, plaques and white stripes associated to multiple red spots, spread over the mucosa or just over the buccal mucosa symmetrically (see **A** and **B**). As it will be obvious from following the diagnostic flowchart, this is the typical appearance of lichen.

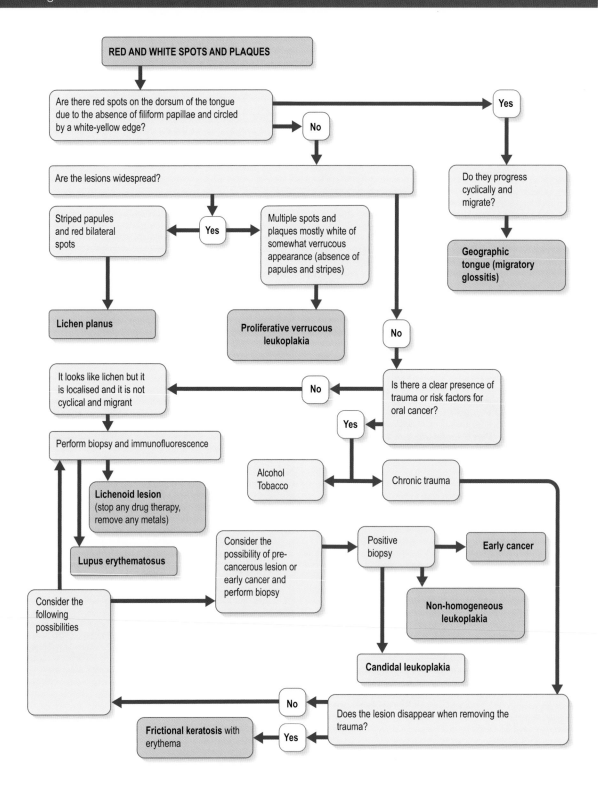

Red Lesions

These lesions are defined by the change of the mucosa, which turns red. An important feature of all these lesions is the epithelium being intact.

Generalised erythema, ecchymoses and petechiae

> If you have observed and recognised red lesions, begin the diagnostic flowchart by selecting one of the following clinical criteria

GENERALISED ERYTHEMA ECCHYMOSES AND PETECHIAE

RED LOCALISED LESIONS (SINGLE OR MULTIPLE)

Red lesions must be differentiated from erosions or ulcers (see further on in this section), which are often red, with loss of tissue. In doubtful cases, examine the lesion after having wiped it thoroughly

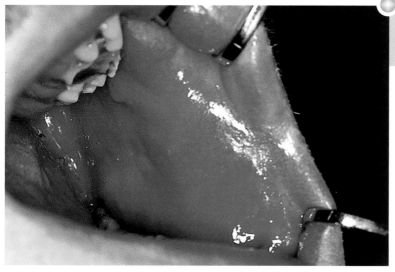

FIGURE 3.9 Generalised erythema is great areas of redness in the oral mucosa that could be spread to all oral sites as in this case.

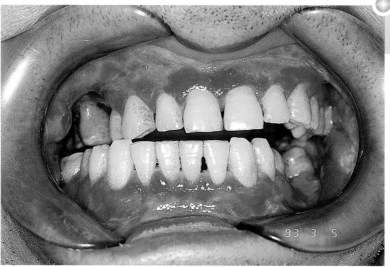

FIGURE 3.10 Generalised erythema may well be localised in one area, such as the gums as it is the case here.

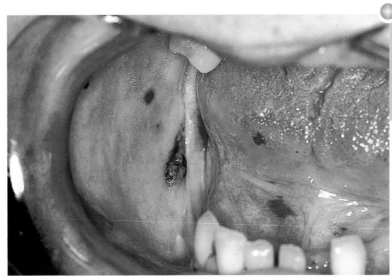

FIGURE 3.11 The **ecchymoses** and **petechiae** are small and widespread red lesions caused by haemorrhage in the mucous membranes. They tend to change colour over time. The difference with small haemangiomas, for which they might be mistaken, is that those do not disappear with vitropression.

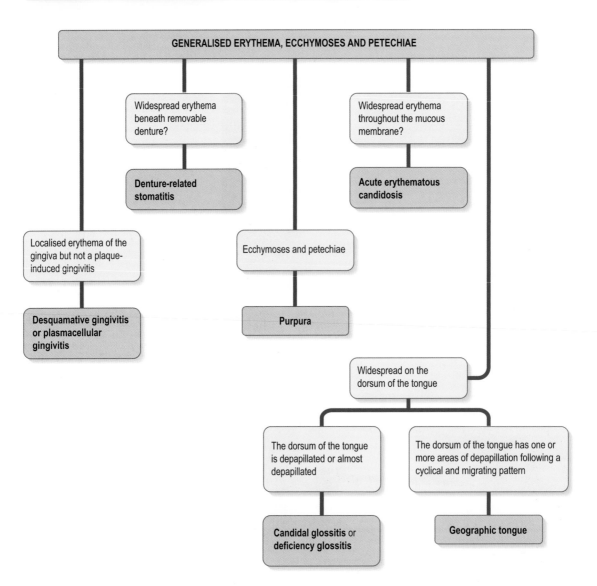

GENERALISED ERYTHEMA, ECCHYMOSES AND PETECHIAE

Widespread erythema beneath removable denture?

Denture-related stomatitis

Localised erythema of the gingiva but not a plaque-induced gingivitis

Desquamative gingivitis or plasmacellular gingivitis

Widespread erythema throughout the mucous membrane?

Acute erythematous candidosis

Ecchymoses and petechiae

Purpura

Widespread on the dorsum of the tongue

The dorsum of the tongue is depapillated or almost depapillated

Candidal glossitis or deficiency glossitis

The dorsum of the tongue has one or more areas of depapillation following a cyclical and migrating pattern

Geographic tongue

Localised red spots (single or multiple)

These are localised and distinguished only by the alteration of colour (genuine spots). If they are slightly on relief (red plaques) or depressed (atrophic), they have the same significance.

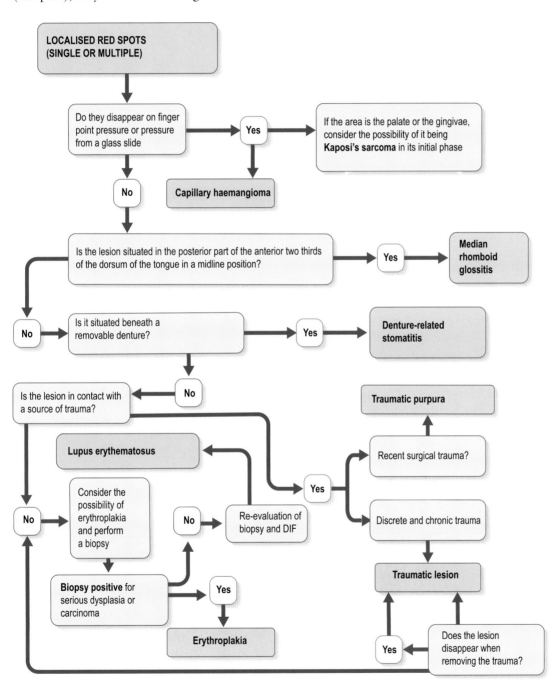

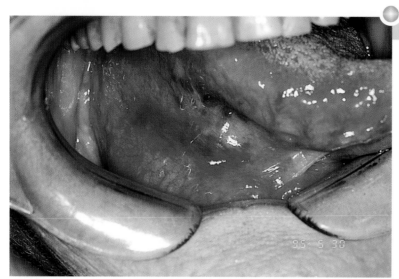

FIGURE 3.12 Single localised red spot.

Erosions

Erosions constitute a superficial loss of epithelium.

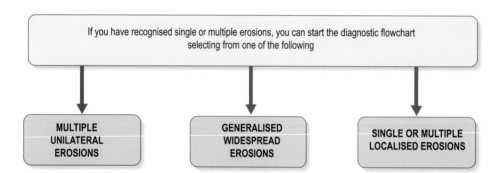

If you have recognised single or multiple erosions, you can start the diagnostic flowchart selecting from one of the following

MULTIPLE UNILATERAL EROSIONS	GENERALISED WIDESPREAD EROSIONS	SINGLE OR MULTIPLE LOCALISED EROSIONS

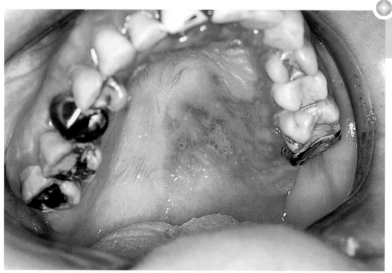

FIGURE 3.13 Multiple unilateral erosions this clinical aspect often points towards some manifestations of herpes.

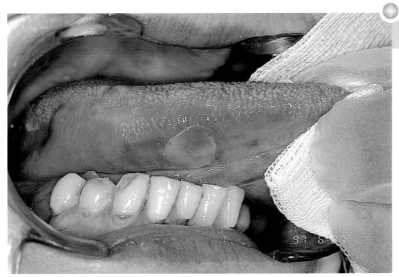

FIGURE 3.14 Single erosions are covered by a yellow layer of fibrin.

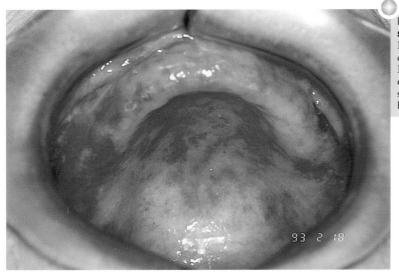

FIGURE 3.15 Generalised wide-spread erosions, with red background. In these cases, it is important to make a differential diagnosis against red spots. Erosions show a clear partial or total loss of the epithelial lining, moreover they are symptomatic (pain and bruising) and may bleed if stimulated.

Note

Note that **erosions** might be the result of previous blisters and vesicles (see below, p. 30).

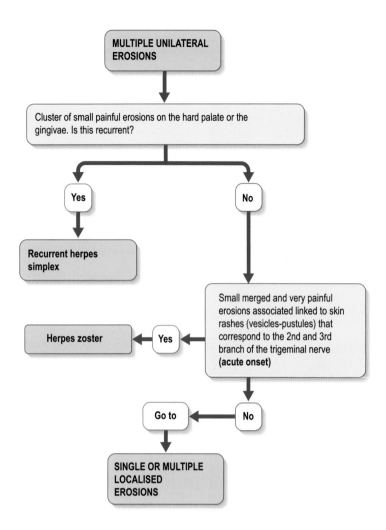

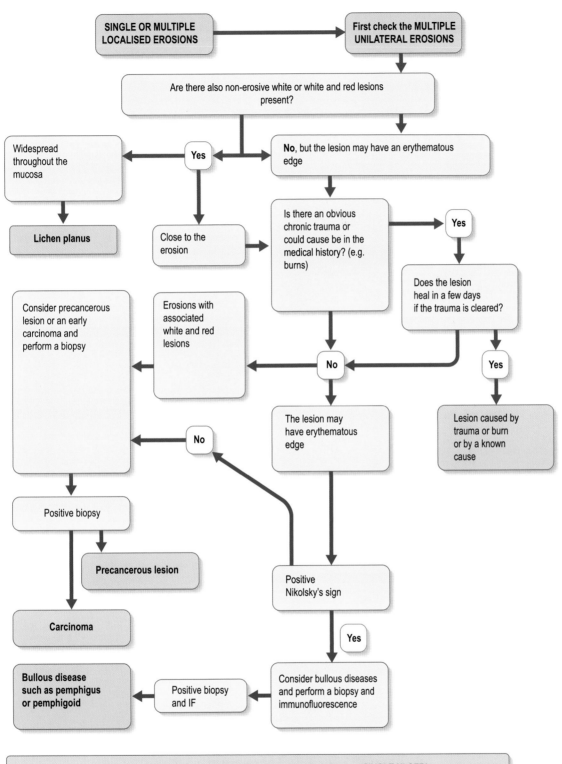

SINGLE OR MULTIPLE LOCALISED EROSIONS → **First check the MULTIPLE UNILATERAL EROSIONS**

Are there also non-erosive white or white and red lesions present?

Yes ← → **No**, but the lesion may have an erythematous edge

Widespread throughout the mucosa → **Lichen planus**

Close to the erosion →

Is there an obvious chronic trauma or could cause be in the medical history? (e.g. burns) → **Yes**

Does the lesion heal in a few days if the trauma is cleared?

Consider precancerous lesion or an early carcinoma and perform a biopsy

Erosions with associated white and red lesions →

No ← **No**

Yes

The lesion may have erythematous edge

Lesion caused by trauma or burn or by a known cause

Positive biopsy →

No →

Precancerous lesion

Carcinoma

Positive Nikolsky's sign

Yes

Bullous disease such as pemphigus or pemphigoid ← Positive biopsy and IF ← Consider bullous diseases and perform a biopsy and immunofluorescence

If in doubt whether these are real erosions or not, please also see 'SINGLE ULCER'

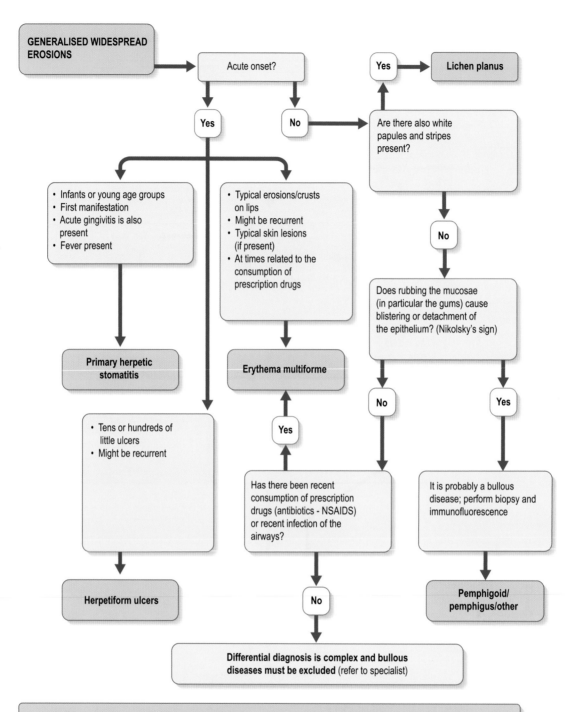

GENERALISED WIDESPREAD EROSIONS

Acute onset?

Yes → **Lichen planus**

Yes

No → Are there also white papules and stripes present?

- Infants or young age groups
- First manifestation
- Acute gingivitis is also present
- Fever present

- Typical erosions/crusts on lips
- Might be recurrent
- Typical skin lesions (if present)
- At times related to the consumption of prescription drugs

No

Does rubbing the mucosae (in particular the gums) cause blistering or detachment of the epithelium? (Nikolsky's sign)

Primary herpetic stomatitis

Erythema multiforme

Yes

No   Yes

- Tens or hundreds of little ulcers
- Might be recurrent

Has there been recent consumption of prescription drugs (antibiotics - NSAIDS) or recent infection of the airways?

It is probably a bullous disease; perform biopsy and immunofluorescence

Herpetiform ulcers   No

Pemphigoid/ pemphigus/other

Differential diagnosis is complex and bullous diseases must be excluded (refer to specialist)

If in doubt about whether these are real erosions or not, please also see "MULTIPLE ORAL ULCERS'

Multiple unilateral erosions

Distinguishing between **erosions** (superficial ulcers) and **ulcers** can be difficult at times, but it is useful because the lesions follow different diagnostic flowcharts.

Ulcers

Ulcers are due to a much deeper loss of tissue than **erosions**: the whole epithelium is breached.

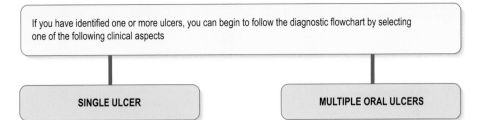

If you have identified one or more ulcers, you can begin to follow the diagnostic flowchart by selecting one of the following clinical aspects

SINGLE ULCER

MULTIPLE ORAL ULCERS

Single ulcer or multiple ulcers

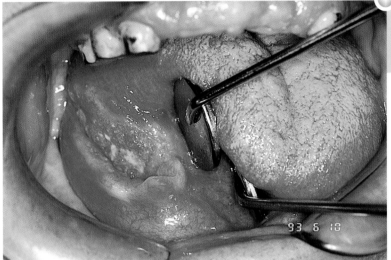

FIGURE 3.16 This neoplastic **single ulcer** constitutes a huge loss of tissue, with a red background (neoplastic tissue) and a yellow area (cellular necrosis and fibrin).

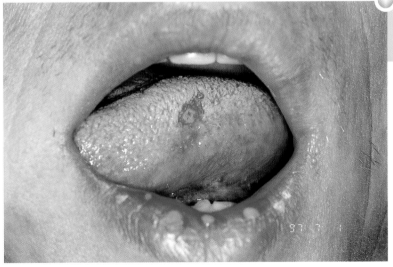

FIGURE 3.17 These **multiple ulcers** of the tongue and the lower lip have typical features, central crater, relieved edges, yellow background (fibrin layer).

Note

Remember that a single ulcer can be oral cancer or another serious oral disease.

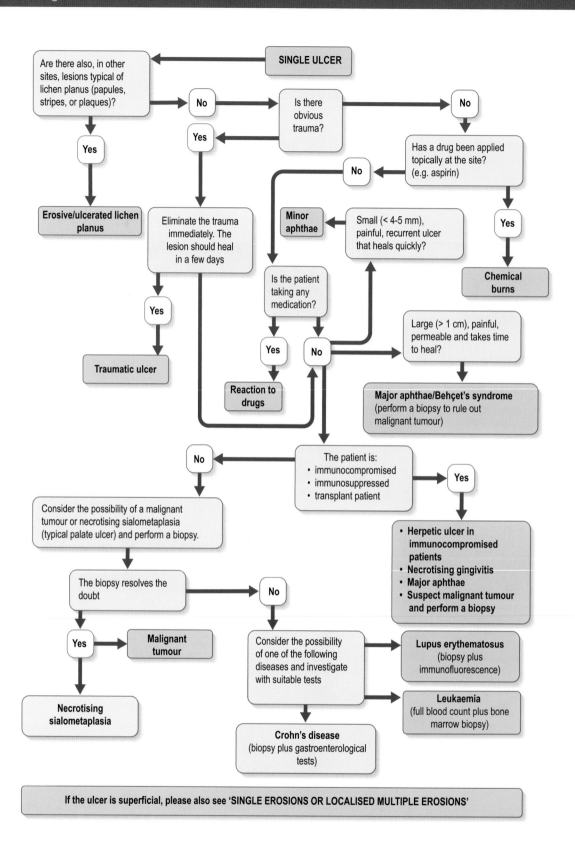

SINGLE ULCER

Are there also, in other sites, lesions typical of lichen planus (papules, stripes, or plaques)?

Is there obvious trauma?

Has a drug been applied topically at the site? (e.g. aspirin)

Erosive/ulcerated lichen planus

Eliminate the trauma immediately. The lesion should heal in a few days

Minor aphthae

Small (< 4-5 mm), painful, recurrent ulcer that heals quickly?

Chemical burns

Is the patient taking any medication?

Large (> 1 cm), painful, permeable and takes time to heal?

Traumatic ulcer

Reaction to drugs

Major aphthae/Behçet's syndrome (perform a biopsy to rule out malignant tumour)

The patient is:
• immunocompromised
• immunosuppressed
• transplant patient

Consider the possibility of a malignant tumour or necrotising sialometaplasia (typical palate ulcer) and perform a biopsy.

• **Herpetic ulcer in immunocompromised patients**
• **Necrotising gingivitis**
• **Major aphthae**
• **Suspect malignant tumour and perform a biopsy**

The biopsy resolves the doubt

Malignant tumour

Consider the possibility of one of the following diseases and investigate with suitable tests

Lupus erythematosus (biopsy plus immunofluorescence)

Necrotising sialometaplasia

Leukaemia (full blood count plus bone marrow biopsy)

Crohn's disease (biopsy plus gastroenterological tests)

If the ulcer is superficial, please also see 'SINGLE EROSIONS OR LOCALISED MULTIPLE EROSIONS'

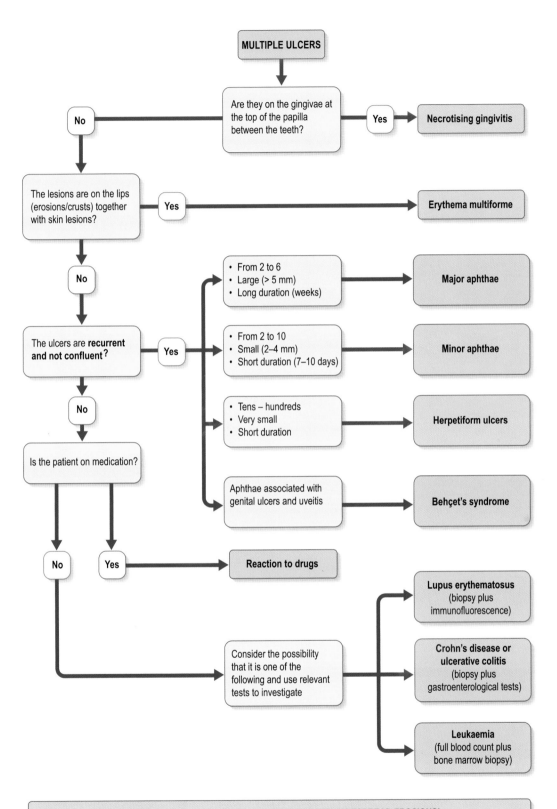

MULTIPLE ULCERS

Are they on the gingivae at the top of the papilla between the teeth? — **Yes** → **Necrotising gingivitis**

No

The lesions are on the lips (erosions/crusts) together with skin lesions? — **Yes** → **Erythema multiforme**

No

The ulcers are **recurrent and not confluent**? — **Yes** →

- From 2 to 6
- Large (> 5 mm)
- Long duration (weeks) → **Major aphthae**

- From 2 to 10
- Small (2–4 mm)
- Short duration (7–10 days) → **Minor aphthae**

- Tens – hundreds
- Very small
- Short duration → **Herpetiform ulcers**

Aphthae associated with genital ulcers and uveitis → **Behçet's syndrome**

No

Is the patient on medication?

- **Yes** → **Reaction to drugs**

- **No** → Consider the possibility that it is one of the following and use relevant tests to investigate →

Lupus erythematosus (biopsy plus immunofluorescence)

Crohn's disease or ulcerative colitis (biopsy plus gastroenterological tests)

Leukaemia (full blood count plus bone marrow biopsy)

If the ulcers are superficial, please also see 'GENERALISED WIDESPREAD EROSIONS'

Blisters and Vesicles

Blisters are lesions consisting of fluid retention within or under the epithelium; they are usually larger than vesicles (from few millimetres to several centimetres). They can be single or multiple but they do not tend to appear in great numbers. **Vesicles** are small pockets of liquid within or under the epithelium. They do not tend to be larger than a few millimetres and the lesions can be numerous (tens, or more).

Blisters

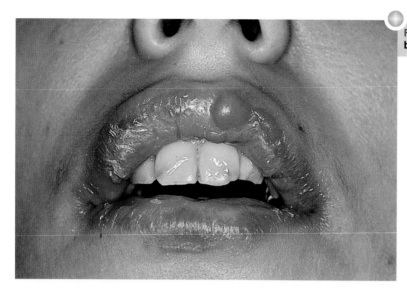

FIGURE 3.18 Serum-filled upper lip **blister.**

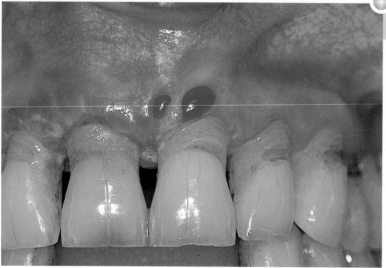

FIGURE 3.19 Two small **blood blisters** on the gingival site.

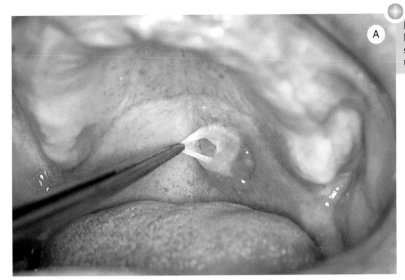

FIGURE 3.20 In the oral cavity **blisters** burst easily giving way to erosions. **(A)** soft palate blister just burst; **(B)** aspect of the same erosion after 2 days.

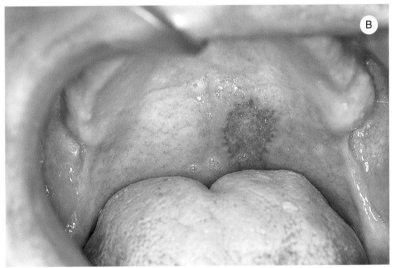

Vesicles

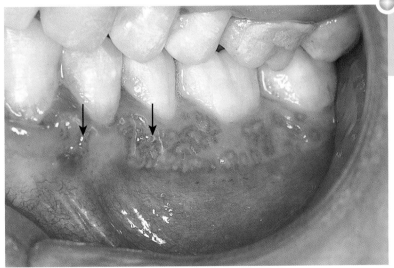

FIGURE 3.21 Vesicles burst easily in the oral cavity giving way to the typical aspect of small multiple confluent erosions. Sometimes, some vesicles remain intact (arrows).

Note

For these lesions follow the diagnostic flowchart for 'Erosions'.

Papillary-verrucous Lesions

Raised lesions on the mucosa can be contained or widespread, they can be sessile or peduncular, white or red, or white and red. They are defined by their thickness (at times this is more than their diameter) and the surface features, which may have some fine digitations or can be chunky.

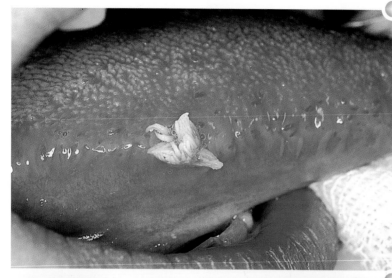

FIGURE 3.22 Typical small white **verrucous lesion** with a small base. They are usually known as pedunculated and they are often benign; in this case representing a papilloma.

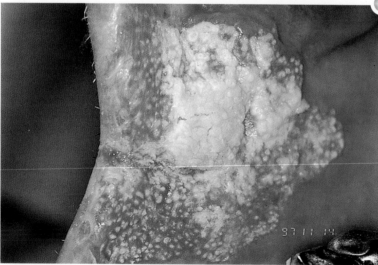

FIGURE 3.23 A large **verrucous lesion** that occupies a larger area. In these lesions, which are called **sessile**, neoplasia is suspected rather strongly. In fact, the case illustrated is a verrucous carcinoma.

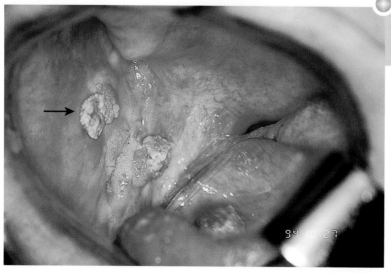

FIGURE 3.24 Not all medium-large verrucous lesions are sessile. The picture shows a small base in a **medium-sized lesion.**

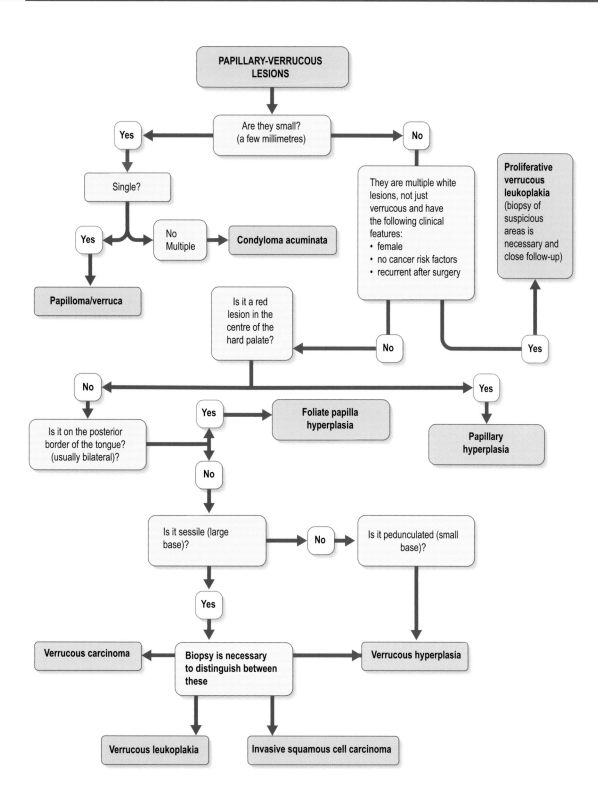

PAPILLARY-VERRUCOUS LESIONS

Are they small? (a few millimetres)

Yes → Single?

Yes → **Papilloma/verruca**

No Multiple → **Condyloma acuminata**

No → They are multiple white lesions, not just verrucous and have the following clinical features:
- female
- no cancer risk factors
- recurrent after surgery

Yes → **Proliferative verrucous leukoplakia** (biopsy of suspicious areas is necessary and close follow-up)

No → Is it a red lesion in the centre of the hard palate?

Yes → **Papillary hyperplasia**

No → Is it on the posterior border of the tongue? (usually bilateral)?

Yes → **Foliate papilla hyperplasia**

No → Is it sessile (large base)?

No → Is it pedunculated (small base)? → **Verrucous hyperplasia**

Yes → **Biopsy is necessary to distinguish between these**

Verrucous carcinoma

Verrucous leukoplakia

Invasive squamous cell carcinoma

Part Two

Clinical features

Chapter Four
Pathology

4

Addison's Disease
(Hypoadrenocorticism)

Clinical features

Oral: Multiple focal spots or diffuse areas of brown pigmentation of buccal mucosae, gingivae, and elsewhere (tongue, lips).

Cutaneous: Hyperpigmentation, especially in sites usually pigmented or traumatised, such as areolae, genitals, flexures.

Incidence

Rare: mainly a disease of young or middle-aged females.

Aetiology

Adrenocortical destruction and subsequent increased release of pituitary adrenocorticotrophic hormone (ACTH), which determines a higher activity of MSH (melanocyte stimulating hormone).

Causes include autoimmune hypoadrenalism and, rarely, tuberculosis, histoplasmosis (sometimes in AIDS), carcinomatosis and Gram-negative sepsis.

Nelson's syndrome is similar, but iatrogenic and results from adrenalectomy in the management of breast cancer.

Diagnosis

Blood pressure, plasma cortisol levels and response to ACTH stimulation (Synacthen test) are all reduced.

Differentiate from other causes of pigmentation, especially racial and drugs.

Management

Replacement therapy (fludrocortisone and corticosteroids). Treat cause.

References

Shah SS, Oh CH, Coffin SE, Yan AC Addisonian pigmentation of the oral mucosa. Cutis 2005 Aug; 76(2):97-99

Lamey PJ, Carmichael F, Scully C Oral pigmentation, Addison's disease and the results of screening for adrenocortical insufficiency. Br Dent J 1985 Apr 20; 158(8):297-298.

Amalgam Tattoo
(Focal argyrosis)

Clinical features

Black or bluish-black (usually) solitary, non-elevated small pigmented area beneath normal mucosa; usually related to lower ridge or buccal vestibule; more rarely palate and floor of the mouth. It is asymptomatic and may rarely be radiopaque.

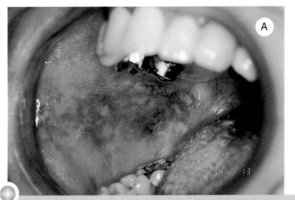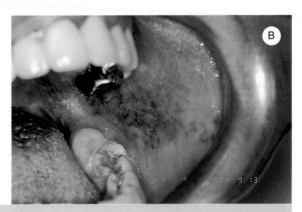

FIGURE 4.1 A & B Oral pigmentation in **Addison's Disease.**

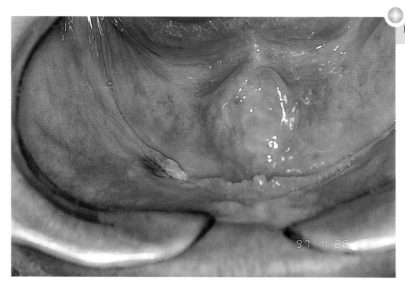

FIGURE 4.2 Amalgam tattoo.

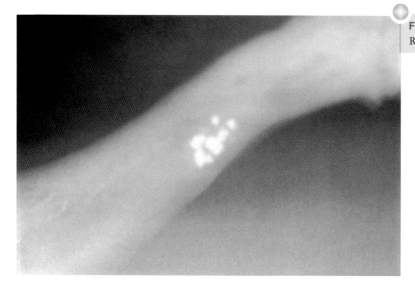

FIGURE 4.3 Amalgam tattoo.
Radiographic appearance of Figure 4.2.

Incidence

Common: mainly in adults.

Aetiology

Amalgam particles or dust can become incorporated in healing wounds after tooth extraction or apicectomy or beneath mucosa (i.e. after an abrasion with a bur or elevator).

Diagnosis

May need to excise to exclude melanoma microscopically.

Differentiate from other causes of pigmentation, especially naevi and melanoma.

Management

The lesions are of no clinical importance but excision biopsy may sometimes be necessary to distinguish reliably from naevus or melanoma, or for aesthetic reasons.

References

Owens BM, Johnson WW, Schuman NJ Oral amalgam pigmentations (tattoos): a retrospective study. Quintessence Int 1992 Dec; 23(12):805-810

Amyloidosis

Clinical features

Macroglossia in up to 50% of patients and oral petechiae or blood-filled bullae.

Incidence

Rare. Oral amyloidosis is almost exclusively primary.

Aetiology

Deposition in tissues of eosinophilic hyaline material with a fibrillar structure on ultramicroscopy.

Deposits are immunoglobulin light chains in primary (usually myeloma-associated or other monoclonal gammopathy) amyloid.

Different proteins are present in secondary and other forms of amyloid. Secondary amyloidosis is now seen mainly in rheumatoid arthritis and ulcerative colitis, and rarely affects the mouth.

Diagnosis

Biopsy, blood picture, ESR and marrow biopsy, serum proteins and electrophoresis, urinalysis (Bences-Jones proteinuria), skeletal survey for myeloma.

Differentiate from other causes of macroglossia, and from other causes of petechiae/bullae, such as localised oral purpura and bleeding tendency.

Management

Treat underlying condition (if myeloma, chemotherapy with melphalan and prednisone).

Surgical reduction of the tongue is inadvisable; tissue is friable, often bleeds excessively and swelling quickly recurs.

References

Koloktronis A, Chatzigiannis I, Paloukidou N Oral involvement in a case of AA amyloidosis. Oral Dis 2003 Sep; 9(5):269-272

Stoor P, Suuronen R, Lindqvist C, Hietanen J, Laine P Local primary (AL) amyloidosis in the palate. A case report. Int J Oral Maxillofac Surg 2004 Jun; 33(4):402-403.

Angina Bullosa Haemorrhagica

Clinical features

Blood-filled blisters mainly on the soft palate and, less commonly, on the tongue borders or in other oral sites. The blisters rapidly develop and on the same day or the next day rupture to leave a non-bleeding ulcer.

Incidence

Not uncommon: mainly in the elderly.

Aetiology

Not defined. Occasionally induced by steroid inhaler.

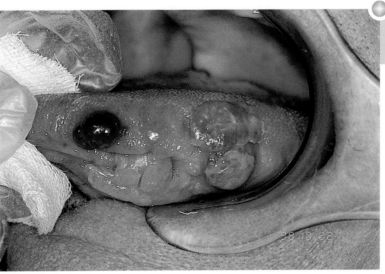

FIGURE 4.4 Oral amyloidosis in a patient with myeloma. Note the macroglossia and the blood filled blister.

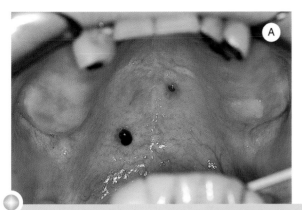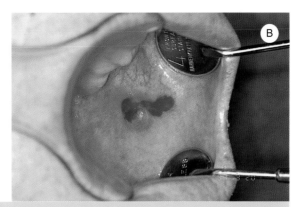

FIGURE 4.5 **Angina bullosa haemorrhagica.** Recently formed blood blisters in the palate (A) and buccal mucosa (B). In both cases there were no coagulation disorders or recent mechanical or thermal trauma.

Diagnosis

Based on the clinical examination and normality of coagulation tests. Biopsy with histological examination and direct immunofluorescence (very rarely necessary) is only carried out in doubtful cases in order to exclude pathologies such as mucous membrane pemphigoid. Differentiate from other causes of oral blisters (pemphigus, pemphigoid, purpura, trauma, burns).

Management

Reassure the patient. Topical analgesics.

References

Deblauwe BM, van der Waal I Blood blisters of the oral mucosa (angina bullosa haemorrhagica). J Am Acad Dermatol 1994 Aug; 31(2, Pt 2):341-344

Giuliani M, Favia GF, Lajolo C, Miani CM Angina bullosa haemorrhagica: presentation of eight new cases and a review of the literature. Oral Dis 2002 Jan; 8(1):54-58

▌Angioedema
(Allergic)

Clinical features

Rapid development of oedematous swelling of lip(s).

Oedema may involve the neck and affect the airway.

Incidence

Uncommon: mainly in those with atopic tendency.

Aetiology

Type 1 allergic response to allergen.

Diagnosis

History of atopic disease and/or exposure to allergen: allergy testing.

Differentiate from other causes of facial swelling.

Management

Mild angioedema: antihistamines.

Severe angioedema: intramuscular adrenaline (epinephrine) and i.v. corticosteroids.

▌Angioedema
(Hereditary)

Clinical features

As in allergic angioedema (above), but precipitated by trauma (e.g. dental treatment). High mortality in some families.

Incidence and aetiology

Rare: genetic defect of inhibitor of activated first component of complement C1 (C1 esterase inhibitor); autosomal dominant inheritance.

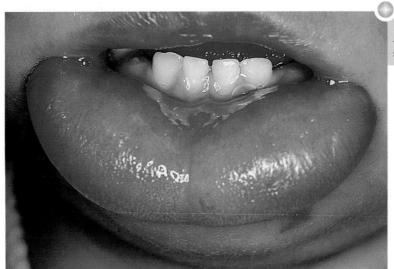

FIGURE 4.6 **Allergic angioedema.**
A severe swelling of the lower lip can be seen.

Diagnosis

Family history. C1 esterase inhibitor and C4 serum levels are low.

Differentiate from other causes of facial swelling.

Management

Stanozolol (an androgenic steroid) or C1 esterase inhibitor.

References

Atkinson JC, Frank MM Oral manifestations and dental management of patients with hereditary angioedema. J Oral Pathol Med 1991 Mar; 20(3):139-142

Karlis V, Glickman RS, Stern R, Kinney L Hereditary angioedema: case report and review of management.Oral Surg Oral Med Oral Pathol Oral Radiol Endod 1997; 83(4):462-464

Rees SR, Gibson J Angioedema and swellings of the orofacial region. Oral Dis 1997; 3(1):39-42

Angular Stomatitis
(Perleche, angular cheilitis)

Clinical features

Symmetrical erythematous fissures on skin of commissures, and (rarely) commissural leukoplakia intraorally.

Incidence

Common: mainly elderly edentulous patients who wear an upper denture.

Aetiology

Usually due to *Candida albicans. Staphylococcus aureus* and/or streptococci may also be cultured from lesions. Most patients have denture-related stomatitis.

Other causes include iron deficiency, hypo-vitaminoses (especially B), malabsorption states (e.g. Crohn's disease), HIV infection, diabetes or other immune defects, antibiotic use, decreased vertical dimension of dentures.

Diagnosis

Clinical. May need blood picture, smears for fungal hyphae and bacteriological culture.

Management

Eliminate any underlying predisposing factors. Treat denture-related stomatitis. Treat angular stomatitis with topical antifungal such as miconazole. Correct vertical dimension, improve oral and denture hygiene, eliminate traumatic factors.

References

Garber GE Treatment of oral Candida mucositis infections. Drugs 1994 May; 47(5):734-740

Porter SR, Scully C Orofacial manifestations in primary immunodeficiencies: T lymphocyte defects. J Oral Pathol Med 1993 Aug; 22(7):308-309

Rogers RS 3rd, Bekic M Diseases of the lips. Semin Cutan Med Surg 1997 Dec; 16(4):328-336

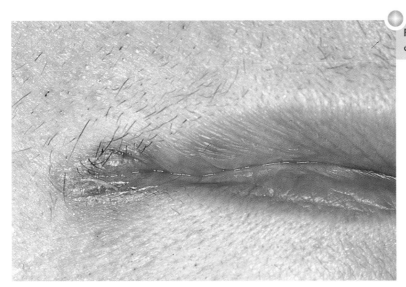

FIGURE 4.7 Angular cheilitis. Typical erythema with fissuring.

Ankyloglossia
(Tongue-tie)

Clinical features
Lingual fraenum anchors tongue tip, restricting protrusion and lateral movements, impairing oral cleansing but rarely interfering with speech. Most cases are partial.

Incidence
Rare, especially complete or lateral ankyloglossia.

Aetiology
May have a genetic basis.

Diagnosis
Clinical. Differentiate from tethering of tongue by scarring, e.g. in epidermolysis bullosa. Tongue-tie is also seen in some rare syndromes.

Management
Surgery (fraenectomy) if severe, if there are speech problems, an inability to lick the lip or to perform internal oral toilet, or if it will interfere with a denture. In rare instances infants have problems with feeding and suction.

References
Kotlow LA Ankyloglossia (tongue-tie): a diagnostic and treatment quandary. Quintessence Int 1999 Apr; 30(4):259-262

Aphthae
(Recurrent aphthous stomatitis - RAS)

Clinical features
Recurrent ulcers. There are three distinct clinical patterns:

Minor: small ulcers (<4 mm) on mobile mucosae (mostly labial and buccal mucosae), less than five ulcers at one time, healing within 14 days, erythematous borders, no vesicle formation, no scarring.

Major: large ulcers (may be >1 cm), any site including dorsum of tongue and hard palate, healing within 1-3 months, with scarring. Extreme pain and lymph node enlargement are common.

Herpetiform ulcers: multiple (10-100), minute (1-2 mm) ulcers that coalesce to produce ragged ulcers. Any part of the oral mucosa, more frequently tip of the tongue, labial mucosa, margins of the tongue.

Incidence
About 25% of population, mostly non-smokers.

Aetiology
Unclear. No reliable evidence of autoimmune disease or any classical immunological reactions. May be cell-mediated immune responses with cross-reactivity between *Streptococcus sanguis*, heat shock protein and oral mucosal tissue.

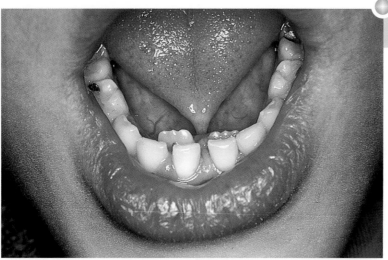

FIGURE 4.8 **Ankyloglossia.** Lingual fraenum impairs the tongue movements.

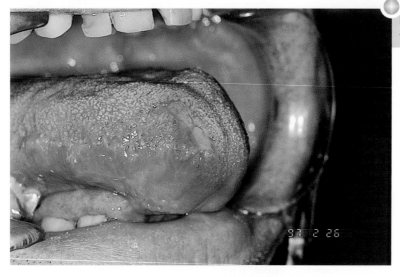

FIGURE 4.9 **Minor aphthae.** Patient with vitamin B_{12} deficiency.

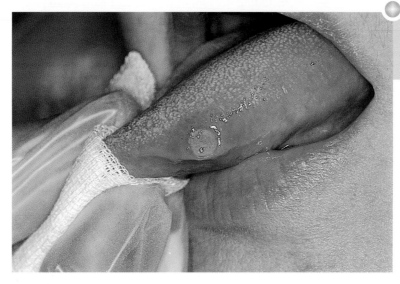

FIGURE 4.10 **Minor aphthae** of the tongue. The ulceration is covered by fibrin and is surrounded by an erythematous border.

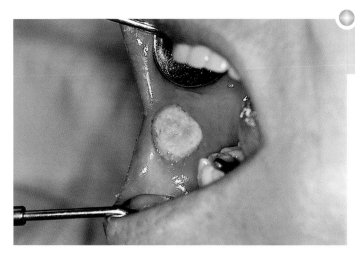

FIGURE 4.11 Major aphthae of the buccal mucosa. The ulcer is > 1 cm in diameter and frequently is long lasting (more than 3 weeks).

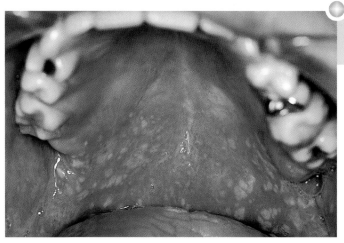

FIGURE 4.12 Herpetiform aphthae of the palate. Several ulcers are evident, bilaterally located and with a tendency to fusion.

Underlying predisposing factors seen in a minority include haematinic deficiency (iron, folate or vitamin B_{12}) in 10-20%, relationship with luteal phase of menstruation (rarely), 'stress', food allergies, HIV disease (major aphthae) and some drugs.

Onset is usually in childhood or adolescence. Later onset may signify haematinic deficiency or HIV disease.

Diagnosis

Diagnosed from history and clinical features. A blood picture is useful to exclude deficiencies. There is no diagnostic test of value.

Differentiate from other causes of mouth ulcers, especially Behçet's syndrome.

Management

Treat any underlying predisposing factors. Treat aphthae with chlorhexidine 0.2% aqueous mouthwash or topical corticosteroids (hydrocortisone hemisuccinate 2.5 mg pellets or 0.1% triamcinolone acetonide in orabase) or tetracycline rinses. Rarely, more potent topical steroids or other agents such as thalidomide may be needed.

References

Jurge S, Kuffer R, Scully C, Porter S VI Recurrent aphthous stomatitis. Oral Dis 2006 Jan; 12(1):1-21

Porter S, Scully C Aphthous ulcers (recurrent). Clin Evid 2004 Jun; (11):1766-1773

Scully C, Gorsky M, Lozada-Nur F Diagnosis and management of recurrent aphthous stomatitis: a consensus approach. J Am Dent Assoc 2003 Feb; 134(2):200-207

Basal Cell Carcinoma
(Basalioma)

Clinical features
Primary basal cell carcinoma occurs only on the skin or on the lips. Manifestations in the oral cavity arise in continuity from facial primary lesions.

It is a slightly translucent, waxy, or pearly papule or nodule, with surrounding or overlying telangiectasia. Secondary changes can include ulceration, crusting, pigmentation and erythema.

It is a slow-growing tumour that metastasizes extremely rarely, although it can be strikingly destructive locally if neglected or inadequately treated.

Aetiology
Predisposing factors include chronic UV exposure, tobacco, chronic radiodermatitis, scars of lupus erythematosus.

Diagnosis
Biopsy is mandatory.

Differentiate from other causes of mouth ulcers or keratoses.

Management
Surgical excision.

References
Rishiraj B, Epstein JB Basal cell carcinoma: what dentists need to know. J Am Dent Assoc 1999 Mar; 130(3):375-380

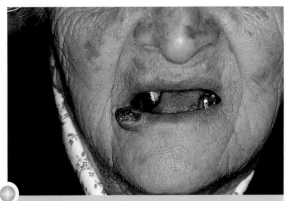

FIGURE 4.13 **Basal cell carcinoma.** Lower lip lesion in an elderly person.

Behçet's Syndrome

Clinical features
Multi-system disorder with ulcers indistinguishable from typical aphthae. Predominantly a disease of adult males.

Oral aphthae: almost invariably.

Genital ulcers: may be muco-cutaneous, usually smaller than oral ulcers.

Eye disease: reduced visual acuity, uveitis, retinal vasculitis, occasionally blindness.

Skin disease: arthralgia of large joints.

Neurological disease: various syndromes.

Others: thromboses, colitis, renal disease, gastrointestinal ulcers, etc.

Incidence
Rare, except in Japan and the Mediterranean region.

Aetiology
Unclear: immunological changes are like those in aphthae. Immune complexes, possibly with herpes simplex virus, may be implicated. Specific but weak HLA associations (B5101).

Diagnosis
Clinical. There is no immunological test of value.

Differentiate from other oculomucocutaneous disorders, especially ulcerative colitis, erythema multiforme, syphilis and Reiter's syndrome.

Management
Systemic: immunosuppression using colchicine, corticosteroids, azathioprine, ciclosporin, dapsone or thalidomide.

Oral ulcers: treat as for aphthae.

References
Al-Otaibi LM, Porter SR, Poate TW Behçet's disease: a review. J Dent Res 2005 Mar; 84(3): 209-222

Sakane T, Takeno M, Suzuki N, Inaba G Behçet's disease. N Engl J Med 1999 Oct 21; 341(17):1284-1291

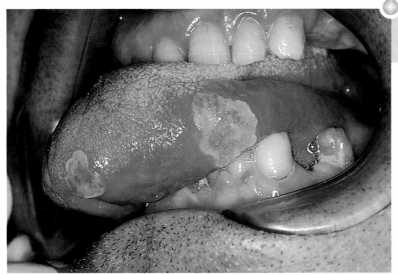

FIGURE 4.14 Behçet's Syndrome. Two aphthous-like ulcers of the tongue are evident.

Scully C, Felix DH Oral medicine; update for the dental practitioner. Mouth ulcers of more serious connotation. Br Dent J 2005 Sep 24; 199(6):339-343

Black or Brown Hairy Tongue

Clinical features
Brown or black hairy appearance of central dorsum of tongue, most severe posteriorly.

Incidence
Uncommon: mainly in middle-aged or older males.

Aetiology
Unknown. Abnormal elongation of filiform papillae. Increased keratin deposition or delayed shedding of cornified layer.

Predisposed by smoking, drugs (e.g. iron salts), dry mouth, chemotherapy, irradiation, oral pH alterations and poor oral hygiene (proliferation of chromogenic microorganisms, not *Candida albicans*).

Diagnosis
Clinical.

Management
Improve oral hygiene; discontinue any drugs responsible; brush tongue (in evenings); suck dry peach stone. In some cases local antifungal or tretinoin therapy may be useful.

References
Langtry JA, Carr MM, Steele MC, Ive FA Topical tretinoin: a new treatment for black hairy tongue (lingua villosa nigra). Clin Exp Dermatol 1992 May; 17(3):163-164

Manabe M, Lim HW, Winzer M, Loomis CA Architectural organization of filiform papillae in normal and black hairy tongue epithelium: dissection of differentiation pathways in a complex human epithelium according to their patterns of keratin expression. Arch Dermatol 1999 Feb; 135(2):177-181

Sarti GM, Haddy RI, Schaffer D, Kihm J Black hairy tongue. J Am Fam Physician 1990 Jun; 41(6): 1751-1755

'Burning Mouth'
(Oral dysaesthesia)

Clinical features
Almost invariably a persistent burning sensation in tongue (occasionally in palate or lip) with no organic disease. Few profess anxiety about cancer or sexually transmitted disease; although some admit this on specific questioning.

Incidence
Common, especially in middle-aged females.

Aetiology
Organic lesions. Deficiency states, erythema migrans, ulcers, lichen planus and candidosis may cause similar symptoms. A normal-appearing

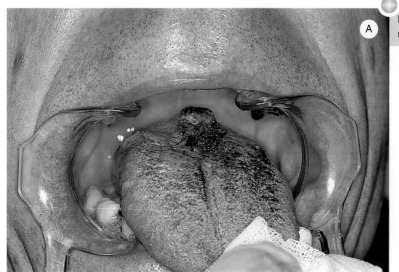

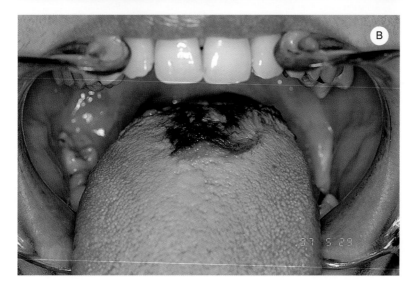

FIGURE 4.15 **Black hairy tongue**, two different patients (A, B).

tongue may be seen in deficiency states, and with psychogenic causes, drugs (e.g. captopril) and diabetes mellitus.

Diagnosis

Blood picture, blood glucose levels; psychiatric investigation for depression.

Differentiate from organic causes.

Management

Treat any organic cause. Otherwise, psychotherapy or antidepressants (usually dothiepin) may be helpful.

References

Bogetto F, Maina G, Ferro G, Carbone M, Gandolfo S Psychiatric comorbidity in patients with burning mouth syndrome. Psychosom Med 1998 May-Jun; 60(3):378-385

Femiano F, Scully C Burning mouth syndrome (BMS): double blind controlled study of alpha-lipoic acid (thioctic acid) therapy. J Oral Pathol Med 2002 May; 31(5):267-916

Maina G, Albert U, Gandolfo S, Vitalucci A, Bogetto F Personality disorders in patients with burning mouth syndrome. J Personal Disord 2005 Feb; 19(1):84-93

Scala A, Checchi L, Montevecchi M, Marini I, Giamberardino MA Update on burning mouth syndrome: overview and patient management. Crit Rev Oral Biol Med 2003; 14(4):275-291

Candidosis
Pseudomembranous candidosis

Clinical features
White or creamy plaques that can be wiped off to leave a red base.

Incidence
Rare in healthy patients.

Aetiology
Neonatal or where oral microflora is disturbed by antibiotics, corticosteroids or xerostomia; immune defects (especially HIV infection), immuno-suppressive management, leukaemias and lymphomas, and diabetes.

Diagnosis
Usually clinical, but Gram stain smear (hyphae) and blood picture may help.

Differentiate from Koplik's or Fordyce's spots and lichen planus.

Management
Treat predisposing cause.

Antifungals: nystatin oral suspension, pastilles, amphotericin lozenges, miconazole gel or tablets, fluconazole tablets.

Erythematous candidosis
Candidosis may cause a sore red mouth, especially in patients on broad spectrum antimicrobials.

Erythematous candidosis, especially on the palate or tongue, may also be a feature of HIV disease.

Chronic mucocutaneous candidosis

Clinical features
Oral: persistent widespread leukoplakia.

Cutaneous: nail and skin candidosis.

Others: rarely familial multiple endocrinopathies.

Incidence
Rare.

Aetiology
Immune defects sometimes identified; occasionally genetic.

Diagnosis
Family history, biopsy, blood picture, auto-antibody and endocrine studies.

Differentiate from other white lesions.

Management
Antifungals.

References
Budtz-Jorgensen E, Lombardi T Antifungal therapy in the oral cavity. Periodontol 2000 1996 Feb; 10:89-106

Cannon RD, Chaffin WL Oral colonization by Candida albicans. Crit Rev Oral Biol Med 1999; 10(3):359-383

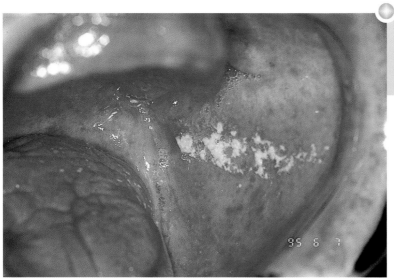

FIGURE 4.16 **Pseudomembranous candidosis** (thrush). On the buccal mucosa there are several white patches composed of hyphae, necrotic material and desquamated epithelium.

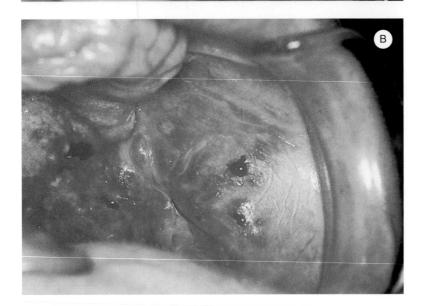

FIGURE 4.17 Pseudomembranous candidosis before (A) and after (B) removal of the patches in a chemo-radio therapy treated patient.

Scully C, el-Kabir M, Samaranayake LP Candida and oral candidosis: a review. Crit Rev Oral Biol Med 1994; 5(2):125-157

Candidal leukoplakia

Clinical features

Candidal leukoplakia is typically found at commissures, often speckled. There is a higher premalignant potential than many leukoplakias.

Incidence

Uncommon.

Aetiology

Unclear aetiology: smoking predisposes.

Diagnosis

Biopsy.

Differentiate from other oral white lesions.

Management

Antifungals, smoking cessation; removal (excision laser or cryosurgery) or observation.

References

Lamey PJ, Lewis MA, MacDonald DG Treatment of candidal leukoplakia with fluconazole. Br Dent J 1989 Apr 22; 166(8):296-298

Sciubba JJ Oral leukoplakia. Crit Rev Oral Biol Med 1995; (2):147-160

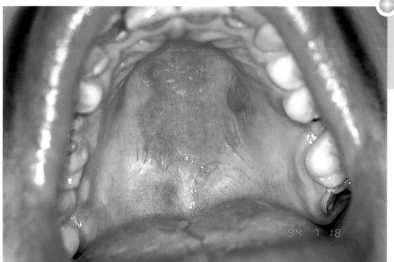

FIGURE 4.18 Erythematous candidosis of the palate. HIV-positive patient with a burning severe erythematous area in the middle of the palate.

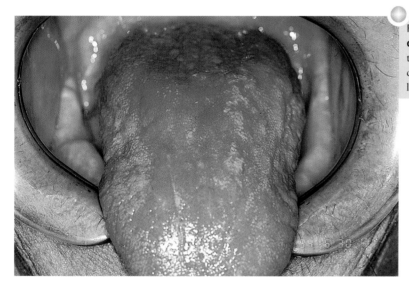

FIGURE 4.19 Erythematous candidosis of the dorsum of the tongue. In this diabetic patient the dorsum of the tongue was reddish with lack of the tongue papillae.

Tradati N, Grigolat R, Calabrese L, et al Oral leukoplakias: to treat or not? Oral Oncol 1997 Sep; 33(5):317-321

Carcinoma, Squamous Cell

Clinical features

On the lip presents with thickening, induration, crusting or ulceration, usually at vermilion border of lower lip. There is late involvement of submental lymph nodes.

Oral cancer sites include the floor of the mouth, ventral and lateral borders of the tongue, retromolar trigone and the soft palate/tonsillar complex.

Early stage oral cancer has numerous and variable clinical appearances. Early lesions can appear as an asymptomatic area with superficial changes to surface colour and texture (red, red-white speckled or white lesions), areas of induration or ulceration, or they may resemble or coexist with common entities, such as candidosis or lichen planus.

In later stages, the clinical appearance is one of an indurated, non-healing ulcer with elevated margins or the neoplasm may have a prominent exophytic as well as an endophytic growth pattern. In this stage, metastases are relatively common.

Incidence

Uncommon: declining on lip, increasing intraorally.

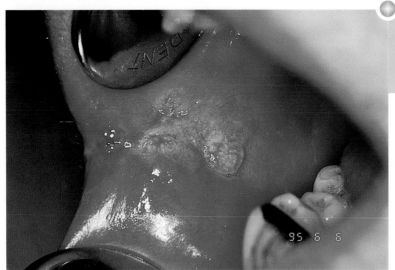

FIGURE 4.20 **Candida leukoplakia** (*see also* Keratosis). On the right retrocommisural area can be seen a non homogeneous-white patch with slight verrucous appearance.

Represent about 4% of all cancers in males and 2% in females.

Aetiology

Predisposing factors include tobacco and alcohol use and, sometimes, UV irradiation (sun). Viruses (HPV) may be involved.

Diagnosis

Biopsy is mandatory.

Differentiate from other causes of mouth ulcers, red lesions or keratoses.

Management

Lip: wedge resection or irradiation. 70% 5-year survival.

Intraoral: surgery or radiotherapy. 30%-40% 5-year survival.

References

Ha PK, Califano JA The role of human papillomavirus in oral carcinogenesis. Crit Rev Oral Biol Med 2004 Jul 1; 15(4):188-196

Mashberg A, Merletti F, Boffetta P, et al Appearance, site of occurrence, and physical and clinical characteristics of oral carcinoma in Torino, Italy. Cancer 1989 Jun 15; 63(12):2522-2527

Petti S, Scully C Oral cancer: the association between nation-based alcohol-drinking profiles and oral cancer mortality. Oral Oncol 2005 Sep; 41(8):828-834

Scully C Oral squamous cell carcinoma; from an hypothesis about a virus, to concern about possible sexual transmission. Oral Oncol 2002 Apr; 38(3): 227-234

Scully C, Bedi R Ethnicity and oral cancer. Lancet Oncol 2000 Sep; 1(1):37-42

Warnakulasuriya S, Sutherland G, Scully C Tobacco, oral cancer, and treatment of dependence. Oral Oncol 2005 Mar; 41(3):244-260

Carcinoma, Verrucous

Clinical features

Lesions typically present as exophytic, cauliflower or wart-like masses, usually associated with leucoplakia. Common on the gingiva, palate, buccal mucosa.

The tumour shows little tendency to lymph node metastasis, but may occasionally change to squamous-cell carcinoma or very aggressive anaplastic carcinoma.

Incidence

This form of carcinoma accounts for 5% of all intraoral squamous cell carcinomas.

Aetiology

Most closely associated with use of tobacco in various forms or HPV.

Diagnosis

Biopsy is mandatory.

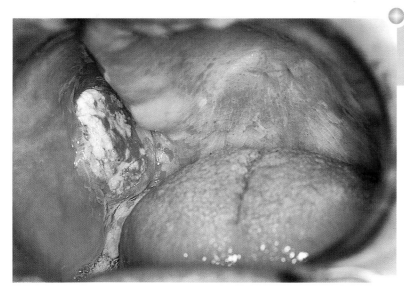

FIGURE 4.21 Squamous cell carcinoma. A buccal mucosal squamous cell carcinoma with features of non-homogeneous leukoplakia.

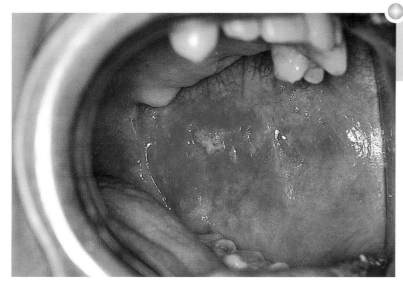

FIGURE 4.22 Squamous cell carcinoma. Early carcinoma of the buccal mucosa with features of a small ulcer within an erythroplasic area.

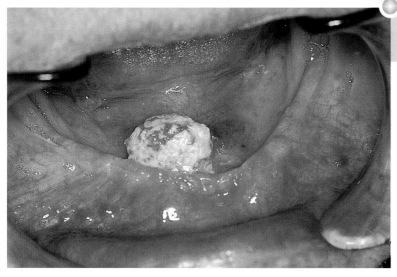

FIGURE 4.23 Squamous cell carcinoma. Exophytic lesion of the floor of the mouth.

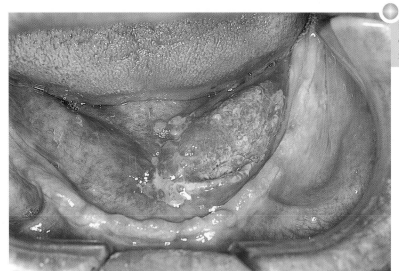

FIGURE 4.24 Squamous cell carcinoma. Ulcerated lesion of the floor of the mouth.

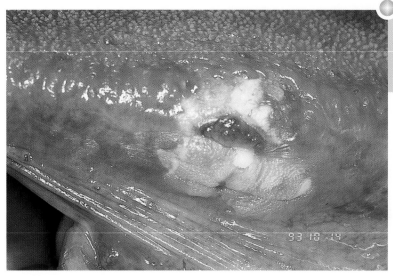

FIGURE 4.25 Squamous cell carcinoma. Early cancer of the border of the tongue with features of a non homogeneous-leukoplakia. Note the central ulceration.

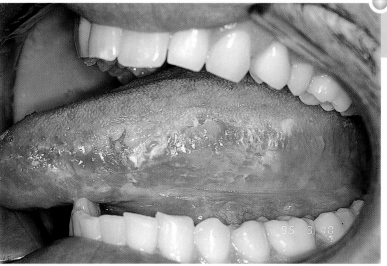

FIGURE 4.26 Non homogeneous-leukoplakia of the border of the tongue. The patient refused treatment.

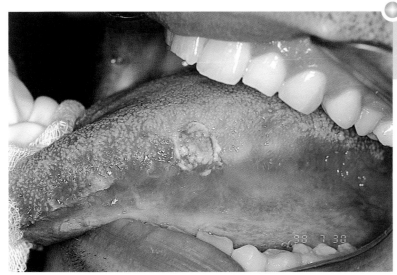

FIGURE 4.27 Squamous cell carcinoma. The same case as Figure 4.26 after 3 years: onset of an early squamous cell carcinoma.

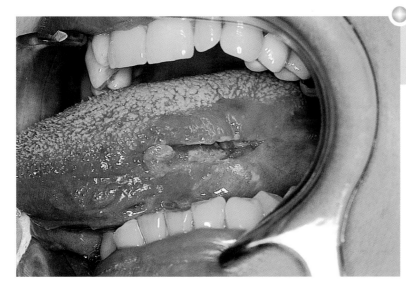

FIGURE 4.28 Squamous cell carcinoma. A deep lingual ulceration. At this stage, lymphadenopathy is frequently found.

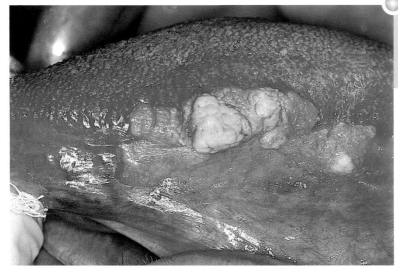

FIGURE 4.29 Squamous cell carcinoma of the border of the tongue. Despite the verrucous-carcinoma appearance, histology showed the invasive nature of the lesion.

Management

The treatment of choice for this cancer is surgery; the prognosis is excellent but local recurrence remains a distinct possibility if inadequate treatment is given.

References

Carrozzo M, Carbone M, Gandolfo S, Valente G, Colombatto P, Ghisetti V An atypical verrucous carcinoma of the tongue arising in a patient with oral lichen planus associated with hepatitis C virus infection. Oral Oncol 1997 May; 33(3):220-225

Ogawa A, Fukuta Y, Nakajima T, Kanno SM, Obara A, Nakamura K, Mizuki H, Takeda Y, Satoh M Treatment results of oral verrucous carcinoma and its biological behavior. Oral Oncol 2004 Sep; 40(8): 793-797

Schwartz RA Verrucous carcinoma of the skin and mucosa. J Am Acad Dermatol 1995 Jan; 32(1):1-21

Cheek Biting

Clinical features

Traumatic abrasion of superficial epithelium leaves whitish fragments on reddish background invariably restricted to lower labial and/or buccal mucosa near occlusal line. No malignant potential.

Incidence

Common.

Aetiology

Anxious personality or anxiety neurosis (*see also* frictional keratosis). Rarely seen in psychiatric disorders (self-mutilation), learning disability or some rare syndromes.

Diagnosis

Clinical.

Differentiate from other causes of white lesions, particularly lichen planus, candidosis and leukoplakia.

Management

Stop the habit, if possible.

If necessary, occlusal splint for prevention.

References

Reichart PA Oral mucosal lesions in a representative cross-sectional study of aging Germans. Community Dent Oral Epidemiol 2000 Oct; 28(5):390-398

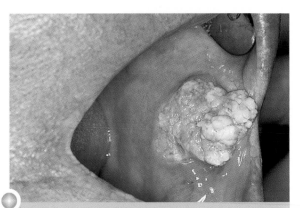

FIGURE 4.30 Verrucous hyperplasia of the buccal mucosa. This benign variety has the same features as verrucous carcinoma.

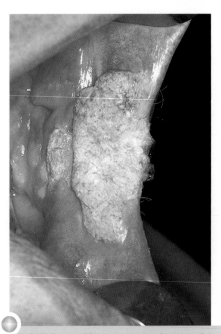

FIGURE 4.31 Verrucous carcinoma of the buccal mucosa. Note the involvement of the commissural area.

Walker RS, Rogers WA Modified maxillary occlusal splint for prevention of cheek biting: a clinical report. J Prosthet Dent 1992 May; 67(5):581-582

Cheilitis
Actinic cheilitis

Clinical features

Erythema, oedema, vesiculation and occasionally haemorrhage; later, whitish lesion or keratosis.

Incidence

Common.

Aetiology

Chronic sun exposure.

Diagnosis

History and clinical features. Biopsy.

Management

Prophylaxis: bland or barrier creams.

References

de Rosa I, Staibano S, Lo Muzio L, Delfino M, Lucariello A, Coppola A, De Rosa G, Scully C Potentially malignant and malignant lesions of the lip. Role of silver staining nucleolar organizer regions, proliferating cell nuclear antigen, p53, and c-myc in differentiation and prognosis. J Oral Pathol Med 1999 Jul; 28(6):252-258

Martinez A, Brethauer U, Rojas IG, Spencer M, Mucientes F, Borlando J, Rudolph MI Expression of apoptotic and cell proliferation regulatory proteins in actinic cheilitis. J Oral Pathol Med 2005 May; 34(5):257-262

Rogers RS 3rd, Bekic M Diseases of the lips. Semin Cutan Med Surg 1997 Dec; 16(4):328-336

Allergic cheilitis

Clinical features

Erythema with fissuring, crusting, desquamation and, therefore, vesicular eruptions on the lips.

In the acute phase slight to severe oedema are seen.

Incidence

Common.

Aetiology

Toothpastes, mouthwashes, dental materials, nail enamel, lipsticks, lip salves, lip liners.

Diagnosis

History and clinical features.

Patch tests.

Differentiate from other causes of cheilitis.

Management

If possible, remove aetiological factors.

References

Gawkrodger DJ Investigation of reactions to dental materials. Br J Dermatol 2005 Sep; 153(3):479-485

Ophaswongse S, Maibach HI Allergic contact cheilitis. Contact Dermatitis 1995 Dec; 33(6): 365-370

Chemical Burns

Clinical features

White lesion with sloughing mucosa localised usually to buccal sulcus and adjacent mucosa, often alongside carious tooth.

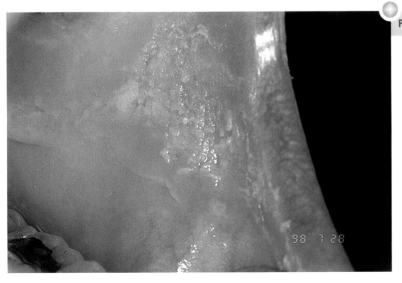

FIGURE 4.32 Frictional keratosis.

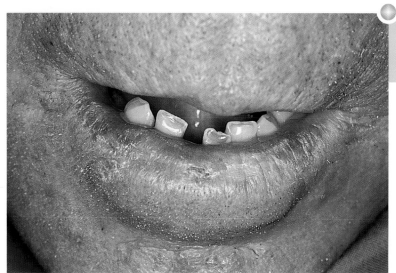

FIGURE 4.33 **Actinic cheilitis.** Owing to the prolonged sun exposure, a cheilitis with red-white patches had developed.

Incidence

Unknown.

Aetiology

Various chemicals or drugs, notably aspirin put in sulcus to try to relieve toothache.

Diagnosis

History and clinical features.

Differentiate from other white lesions.

Management

Treat toothache as appropriate. Stop the habit: lesion is self-healing (usually within 14 days).

References

Moghadam BK, Gier R, Thurlow T Extensive oral mucosal ulcerations caused by misuse of a commercial mouthwash. Cutis 1999 Aug; 64(2):131-134

Scully C, Porter S Orofacial disease: update for the dental clinical team: 3. White lesions. Dent Update 1999 Apr; 26(3):123-129

▌Cracked Lip

Clinical features

Single, persistent painful vertical fissure that bleeds on stretching the lip and opening the mouth wide.

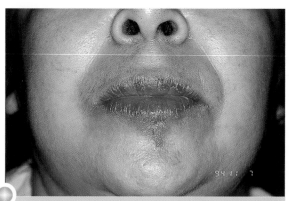

FIGURE 4.34 **Allergic cheilitis.** Note the reddish appearance and the desquamation involving both of the lips.

Incidence and aetiology

Common during cold, windy, winter weather.

Diagnosis

History and clinical features.

Differentiate from angular stomatitis.

Management

Prophylaxis: bland or barrier creams.

References

Kuffer R, Husson C Superficial cheilitis and angular cheilitis. Ann Dermatol Venereol 2000 Jan; 127(1):88-92

Rogers RS 3rd, Bekic M Diseases of the lips. Semin Cutan Med Surg 1997; 16(4):328-336

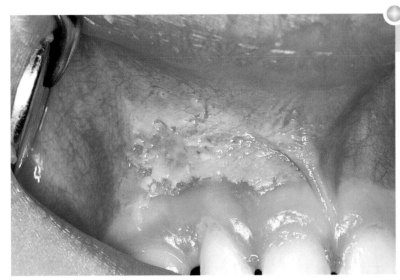

FIGURE 4.35 **Chemical burn** caused by chlorhexidine.

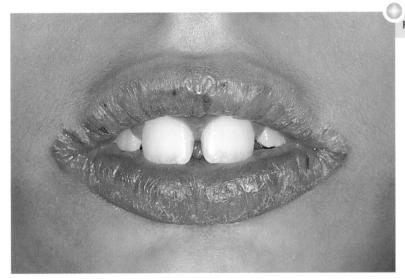

FIGURE 4.36 **Cracked lips.**

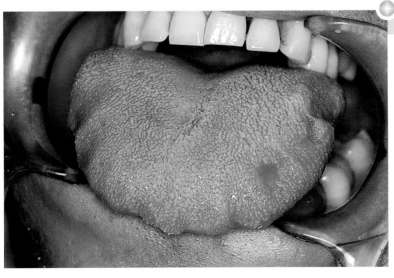

FIGURE 4.37 **Crenated tongue.**

Crenated Tongue

Clinical features

Shallow impressions on the margins of the tongue due to to the neighbouring teeth.

Incidence

Common.

Aetiology

Frequent in macroglossia, bruxism and in persons who are chronically anxious or have the habit of pressing the tongue hard against the teeth.

Diagnosis

History and clinical features.

Differentiate from causes of macroglossia.

Management

Reassurance.

Crohn's Disease

Clinical features

Ulcers, typically solitary, persistent and ragged with hyperplastic margins. May be facial swelling, mucosal tags or cobblestoning.

Incidence

Uncommon.

Aetiology

Unknown.

Diagnosis

Biopsy; full blood picture; gastrointestinal and immunological studies if necessary.

Differentiate from other causes of mouth ulcers, especially malignant lesions or chronic bacterial infections.

Management

Topical or intralesional corticosteroids; systemic or possibly topical sulfasalazine.

References

Harty S, Fleming P, Rowland M, Crushell E, McDermott M, Drumm B, Bourke B A prospective study of the oral manifestations of Crohn's disease. Clin Gastroenterol Hepatol 2005 Sep; 3(9):886-891

Leao JC, Hodgson T, Scully C, Porter S Review article: orofacial granulomatosis. Aliment Pharmacol Ther 2004 Nov; 20(10):1019-1027

Pittock S, Drumm B, Fleming P, McDermott M, Imrie C, Flint S, Bourke B The oral cavity in Crohn's disease. J Pediatr 2001 May; 138(5):767-771

Denture-Induced Hyperplasia
(Denture granuloma or epulis fissuratum)

Clinical features

Usually seen in the buccal sulcus as a painless lump parallel to alveolar ridge with a smooth pink surface. May be grooved by denture margins. Usually related to lower complete denture, especially anteriorly.

Incidence

Common: mainly in middle-aged or elderly patients.

Aetiology

Pressure from denture flange causes chronic irritation and hyperplastic response.

Diagnosis

Usually the diagnosis is clearcut if the lesion is in relation to denture flange. If ulcerated, it may mimic carcinoma (rarely).

Management

Relieve denture flange to prevent recurrence. Surgical removal of hyperplastic tissue may be necessary.

References

Esmeili T, Lozada-Nur F, Epstein J Common benign oral soft tissue masses. Dent Clin North Am 2005 Jan; 49(1):223-240

Macedo Firoozmand L, Dias Almeida J, Guimaraes Cabral LA Study of denture-induced fibrous hyperplasia cases diagnosed from 1979 to 2001. Quintessence Int 2005 Nov-Dec; 36(10):825-829

Thomas GA Denture-induced fibrous inflammatory hyperplasia (epulis fissuratum): research aspects. Aust Prosthodont J 1993; 7:49-55

Wright SM, Scott BJ Prosthetic assessment in the treatment of denture hyperplasia. Br Dent J 1992 Apr 25; 172(8):313-315

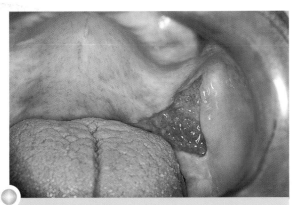

FIGURE 4.38 **Crohn's disease.** Large irregular ulceration.

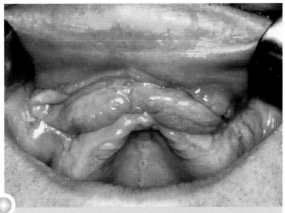

FIGURE 4.40 **Epulis fissuratum** (denture-induced fibrous hyperplasia).

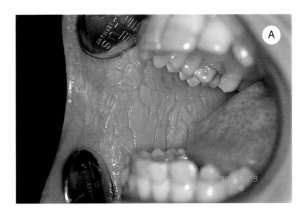

A

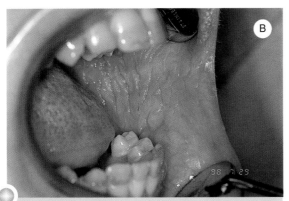

B

FIGURE 4.39 **Crohn's disease (A, B).** Cobblestone appearance of the bilateral buccal mucosae resembling fissured tongue.

Denture-Related Stomatitis

Clinical features

Diffuse erythema of denture-bearing area only, with occasional petechiae. It is almost always asymptomatic. Complications include angular stomatitis and aggravation of palatal papillary hyperplasia.

Incidence

Common (up to 60% of denture wearers): mainly elderly patients.

Aetiology

Usually *C. albicans.* Constant denture-wearing predisposes, but other factors may include poor denture hygiene, high carbohydrate diet and HIV infection.

Diagnosis

Diagnosis is clearcut; smear for hyphae.

Differentiate from erythroplasia or trauma.

Management

Leave dentures out at night in anti-fungal (e.g. hypochlorite, chlorhexidine), give antifungals, attention to dentures.

References

Koray M, Ak G, Kurklu E Fluconazole and/or hexetidine for management of oral candidiasis associated with denture-induced stomatitis. Oral Dis 2005 Sep; 11(5):309-313

Scully C, Felix DH Oral medicine-update for the dental practitioner: red and pigmented lesions. Br Dent J 2005 Nov 26; 199(10):639-645

Yildirim MS, Hasanreisoglu U, Hasirci N, Sultan N Adherence of Candida albicans to glow-discharge modified acrylic denture base polymers. J Oral Rehabil 2005 Jul; 32(7):518-525

■Desquamative Gingivitis

Not a disease entity but a clinical term for persistently sore, glazed and red or ulcerated gingivae.

Incidence

Fairly common: almost exclusively a disease of middle-aged or elderly females.

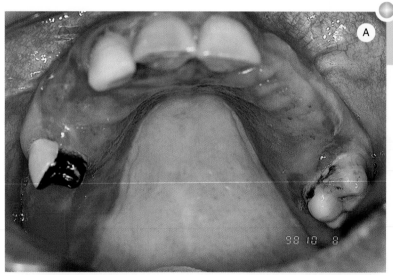

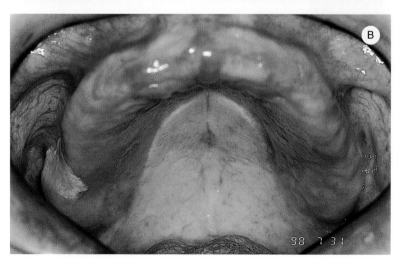

FIGURE 4.41 **Denture related stomatitis.** Diffuse erythema of denture-bearing area (A, B).

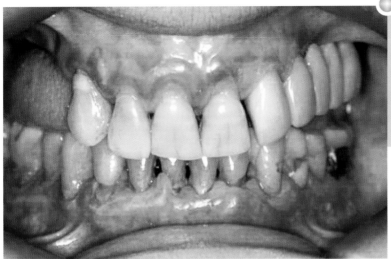

FIGURE 4.42 Desquamative gingivitis (*see also* Lichen planus, Pemphigus vulgaris, Mucous membrane pemphigoid). Diffuse redness of upper and lower vestibular gingiva; the mucosa is fragile and can be easily stripped away. Note the close resemblance of this gingival lichen planus with the gingiva in pemphigoid shown in Figure 4.43.

Aetiology

Usually a manifestation of atrophic lichen planus or mucous membrane pemphigoid.

Occasionally seen in pemphigus or other dermatoses (dermatitis herpetiformis, linear IgA disease) or drugs/chemicals (sodium lauryl sulphate).

Clinical features

Gingivae are red and glazed, sometimes ulcerated, patchily or uniformly, especially labially.

Gingival margins and edentulous ridges tend to be spared.

Erythema is exaggerated where oral hygiene is poor.

Other oral or cutaneous lesions of dermatoses may be associated.

Nikolsky's sign may be positive.

Diagnosis

Biopsy and immunofluorescence.

Differentiate mainly from acute candidosis and chronic marginal gingivitis.

Management

Improve oral hygiene; topical corticosteroids, tacrolimus or dapsone.

Corticosteroids creams used overnight in a polythene splint may help.

References

Jordan RC Diagnosis of periodontal manifestations of systemic diseases. Periodontol 2000 2004; 34:217-229

Robinson NA, Wray D Desquamative gingivitis: a sign of mucocutaneous disorders: a review. Aust Dent J 2003 Dec; 48(4):206-211

Scully C, Carrozzo M, Gandolfo S, Puiatti P, Monteil R Update on mucous membrane pemphigoid: a heterogeneous immune-mediated subepithelial blistering entity. Oral Surg Oral Med Oral Pathol Oral Radiol Endod 1999 Jul; 88(1):56-68

▌Drug-Induced Hyperpigmentation

Clinical features

Variable colour, patchy or localised according to cause.

Incidence

Rare.

Aetiology

A variety of drugs rarely cause pigmentation, and often by unknown mechanisms. Adrenocorticotrophic hormone (ACTH) can cause pigmentation by virtue of melanocyte-stimulating hormone-like activity (ACTH-producing neoplasms act similarly). In the past, heavy metals (e.g. lead) caused pigmented lines due to sulphide deposits in gingival pockets. Drugs currently implicated include anti-malarials,

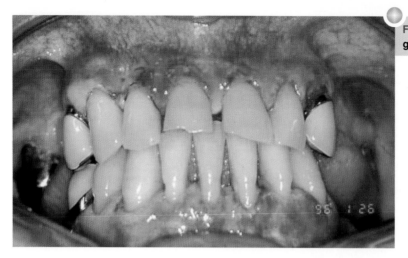

FIGURE 4.43 Desquamative gingivitis in a patient with pemphigoid.

busulfan, cisplatin, phenothiazines, ACTH, zidovudine, minocycline and oral contraceptives.

Diagnosis

History of exposure to drug.

Differentiate from other causes of pigmentation.

Management

Stop the causative drug if possible.

References

Kleinegger CL, Hammond HL, Finkelstein MW Oral mucosal hyperpigmentation secondary to antimalarial drug therapy. Oral Surg Oral Med Oral Pathol Oral Radiol Endod 2000 Aug; 90(2):189-194

Sanchez AR, Rogers RS 3rd, Sheridan PJ Tetracycline and other tetracycline-derivative staining of the teeth and oral cavity. Int J Dermatol 2004 Oct; 43(10):709-715

Scully C Drug-induced oral mucosal hyperpigmentation. Prim Dent Care 1997; 4(1):35-36

Scully C, Felix DH Oral medicine: update for the dental practitioner: red and pigmented lesions. Br Dent J 2005 Nov 26; 199(10):639-645

Drug-Induced Lesions

Clinical features

Cytotoxic induced ulcers: non-specific.

Lichenoid lesions: resemble lichen planus clinically and histologically.

Chemical burns: usually solitary lesions with sloughing of mucosa.

Erythema multiforme: ulcers and lip swelling.

Incidence

Ulcers are common in those on cytotoxic drugs. Other reactions are uncommon or rare.

Aetiology

A wide spectrum of drugs can occasionally cause mouth lesions, by various mechanisms. The more common examples include:

- Cytotoxic agents, particularly methotrexate, producing ulcers.
- Agents producing lichen-planus-like (lichenoid) lesions, such as antihypertensives, antidiabetics, gold salts, non-steroidal antiinflammatory agents, antimalarials and other drugs.
- Agents causing local chemical burns (especially aspirin held in the mouth).
- Agents causing erythema multiforme (especially sulphonamides and barbiturates).

Diagnosis

Drug history: test effect of withdrawal.

Management

Stop causative drug; symptomatic.

References

Guggenheimer J Oral manifestations of drug therapy. Dent Clin North Am 2002 Oct; 46(4):857-868

Korstanje MJ Drug-induced mouth disorders. Review. Clin Exp Dermatol 1995 Jan; 20(1):10-18

Scully C, Bagan JV Adverse drug reactions in the orofacial region. Crit Rev Oral Biol Med. 2004 Jul 1; 15(4):221-239

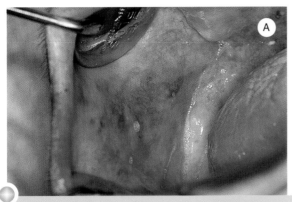
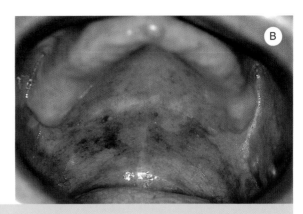
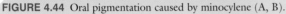

FIGURE 4.44 Oral pigmentation caused by minocylene (A, B).

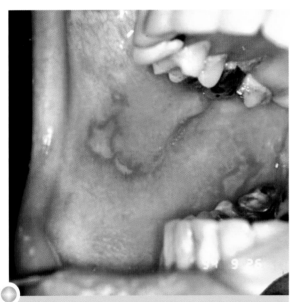

FIGURE 4.45 **Drug-induced lesions.** Erosion/ulcers caused by ketoprofen (an NSAID).

Epulis

Epulides are localised gingival swellings and rarely true neoplasms.

Clinical features

Painless, exophytic, nodular mass usually pedunculated with a smooth or lobulated surface. The colour should be the same as the surrounding gingiva (fibrous epulis) or deep red (pyogenic/pregnancy granuloma) or purple-blue (giant cell granuloma).

Incidence

Common.

Aetiology

Local gingival irritation caused by calculus. Giant cell epulides may result from proliferation of giant cell persisting after resorption of deciduous teeth.

Diagnosis

Excision biopsy, radiography.

Management

Excision; remove irritants. Pregnancy epulides should be preferably excised post-partum if they persist.

References

Binnie WH Periodontal cysts and epulides. Periodontol 2000. 1999 Oct; 21:16-32

Coventry J, Griffiths G, Scully C, Tonetti M ABC of oral health: periodontal disease. BMJ 2000 Jul; 321(7252):36-39

Esmeli T, Lozada-Nur F, Epstein J Common benign oral soft tissue masses. Dent Clin North Am 2005 Jan; 49(1):223-240

Other Gingival Hyperplasia

Crohn's disease

See above.

Drug-induced

Ciclosporin, nifedipine and phenytoin are the most frequent drugs involved.

Gingival fibromatosis

Usually enlarged maxillary tuberosities are present. Less common are generalised gingival

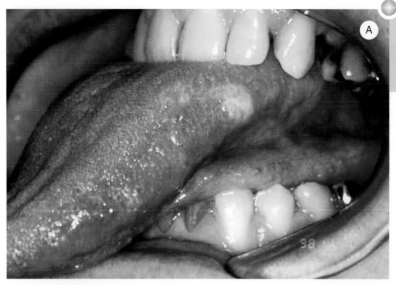

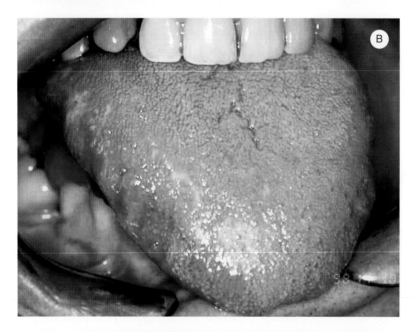

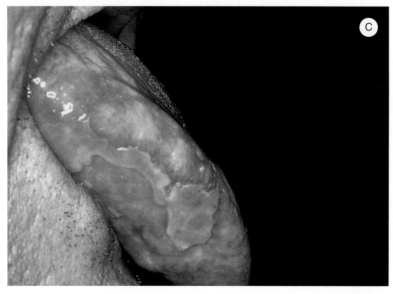

FIGURE 4.46 Drug-induced lesions.
Plaque-like lichenoid lesions of the border and dorsum of the tongue (A, B) and severe lingual erosions (C), all caused by allopurinol.

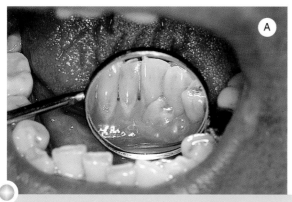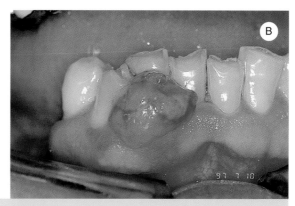

FIGURE 4.47 Pyogenic granuloma (epulis) (A, B). These exophytic masses may have variable dimension, deep-red or purple-blue colour, soft consistency and they bleed easily.

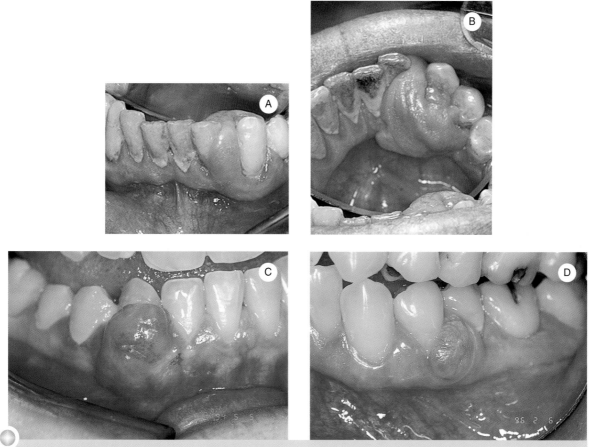

FIGURE 4.48 Fibrous epulis. (A) Vestibular aspect of a fibrous epulis. (B) Lingual appearance of (A). (C) Sometime a red appearance may be seen and, mainly, in the early stage, the gingival swelling may be modest (D).

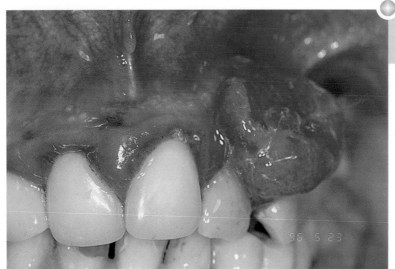

FIGURE 4.49 Pregnancy granuloma.
This epulis developed at third trimester of pregnancy.

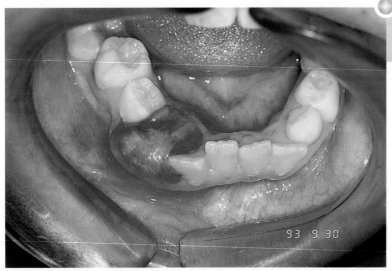

FIGURE 4.50 Gigantocellular epulis.
In this 10-year-old female the onset of the epulis caused the missing 8.3.

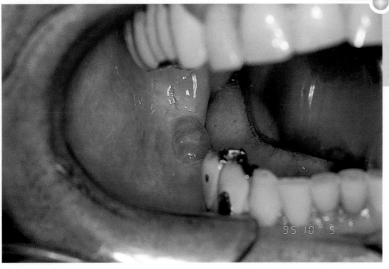

FIGURE 4.51 Gigantocellular epulis remains after the extraction of 4.7. This kind of epulis does not heal with the simple extraction of the tooth involved; careful bone curettage is needed.

hyperplasia or posterior mandibular fibromatosis. The hereditary gingival fibromatoses are often associated with hirsutism. Rarely, the fibromatosis is one feature of a syndrome.

Malignant diseases

Carcinoma of the gingiva is uncommon but possible. Rare secondary localisation may mimic simple epulides, but often are sessile and larger than epulides. Occasionally, Kaposi's sarcoma affect gingiva in AIDS patients.

Wegener's granulomatosis

Can present an almost pathognomonic 'strawberry' appearance of gingiva. There may be lung and kidney lesions and serum antineutrophil cytoplasmic antibodies (ANCA).

Management

Treatment of underlying predisposing condition if possible. In drug-induced hyperplasias, stop causative drug if possible and surgery. Chlorexidine mouthwashes are helpful.

If systemic disease refer to a specialised centre.

References

Camargo PM, Melnick PR, Pirih FQ, Lagos R, Takei HH Treatment of drug-induced gingival enlargement: aesthetic and functional considerations. Periodontol 2000 2001;27:131-138

Garzino-Demo P, Carbone M, Carrozzo M, Broccoletti R, Gandolfo S An increase in gingival volume induced by drugs (phenytoin, cyclosporine and calcium antagonists). A review of the literature. Minerva Stomatol 1998 Sep; 47(9):387-398

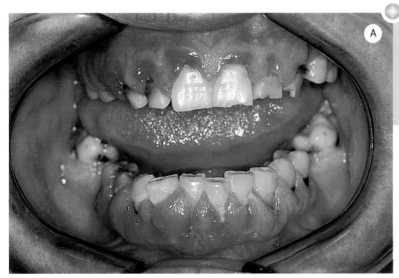

A

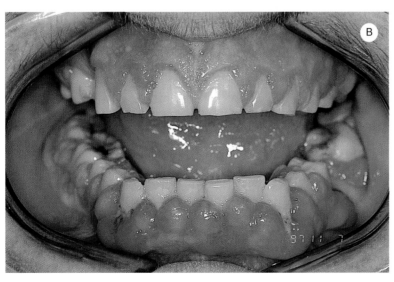

B

FIGURE 4.52 Drug-induced gingival swelling. Chronic intake of drugs such as ciclosporin in organ-transplant patients (A, B) or calcium antagonists (mainly nifedipine) in patients with hypertension (C) causes gingival swelling within 3 months.

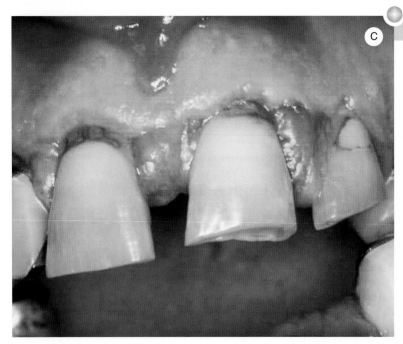

FIGURE 4.52 *Continued.*

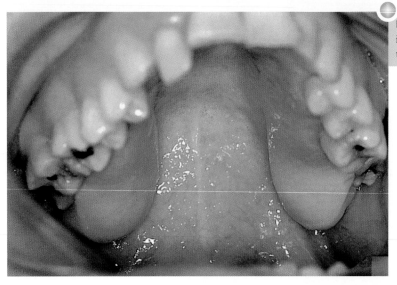

FIGURE 4.53 Gingival fibromatosis involving mainly the maxillary tuberosities, asymmetrically enlarged.

Gomez D, Faucher A, Picot V, Siberchicot F, Renaud-Salis JL, Bussieres E, Pinsolle J Outcome of squamous cell carcinoma of the gingiva: a follow-up study of 83 cases. J Craniomaxillofac Surg 2000 Dec; 28(6):331-335

Periodontal diseases. Lancet 2005 Nov 19; 366(9499):1809-1820

Pihlstrom BL, Michalowicz BS, Johnson NW Periodontal diseases. Lancet 2005 Nov 19; 366(9499):1809-1820

Ponniah I, Shaheen A, Shankar KA, Kumaran MG Wegener's granulomatosis: the current understanding. Oral Surg Oral Med Oral Pathol Oral Radiol Endod 2005 Sep; 100(3):265-270

Erythema Migrans
(Benign migratory glossitis, geographic tongue)

Clinical features

Often asymptomatic, occasionally sore areas on the tongue, especially with acidic foods (e.g. tomatoes). There are irregular, pink or red depapillated areas, sometimes surrounded by distinct yellowish slightly raised margins, which change in shape, increase in size, and spread or move to other areas within hours. It typically involves the dorsum and lateral borders of the

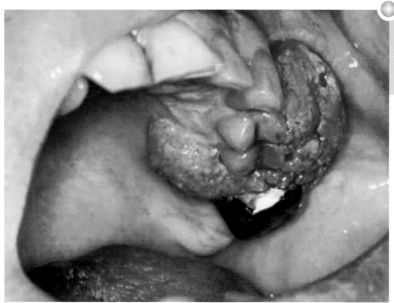

FIGURE 4.54 Squamous cell carcinoma of the gingiva. Very rarely a squamous cell carcinoma may resemble an inflammatory gingival swelling, as in this photograph.

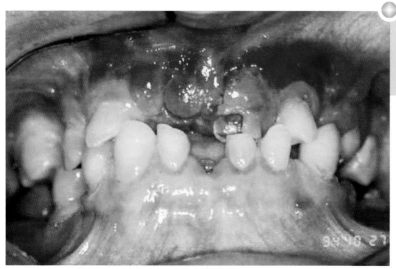

FIGURE 4.55 Kaposi's sarcoma of the gingiva in an HIV-positive patient. On the maxillary gingiva there is a red-brown swelling looking like a gigantocellular epulis.

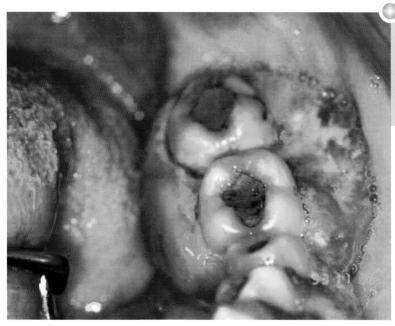

FIGURE 4.56 Non-Hodgkin lymphoma of the gingiva in an HIV-positive patient. This patient had a mandibular gingival swelling clinically diagnosed as epulis. The diagnosis of HIV infection was made after the diagnosis of oral lymphoma.

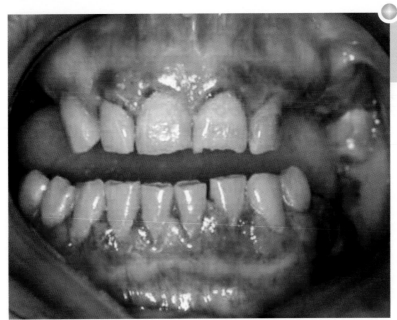

FIGURE 4.57 Wegener granulomatosis. Upper and lower gingivae have the pathognomonic 'strawberry' appearance.

tongue, and rarely adjacent or other oral mucosae. The tongue is often also fissured. The condition may persist for months or years: remissions and recurrences may be present.

Incidence

Common: 1-2% of adults.

Aetiology

Genetic. Associated with psoriasis in 4%.

Diagnosis

Clinical.

Very similar lesions may be seen in psoriasis and Reiter's syndrome (transiently). There also may be confusion with lichen planus and lupus erythematosus.

Management

Reassure. In symptomatic patients, topical steroids or anaesthetics.

References

Gonzaga HF, Torres EA, Alchorne MM, Gerbase-Delima M Both psoriasis and benign migratory glossitis are associated with HLA-Cw6. Br J Dermatol 1996 Sep; 135(3):368-370

Jainkittivong A, Langlais RP Geographic tongue: clinical characteristics of 188 cases. J Contemp Dent Pract 2005 Feb 15; 6(1):123-135

Scully C, Felix DH Oral medicine: update for the dental practitioner: red and pigmented lesions. Br Dent J 2005 Nov 26; 199(10):639-645

Erythema Multiforme

Clinical features

Recurrent attacks, for 10-14 days once or twice a year, of lesions affecting mouth alone, or skin and/or other mucosae. The minor form affects only one site.

- *Oral*: cracked, bleeding, crusted, swollen lips and ulcers. Buccal mucosa, tongue and palate may be involved.
- *Others*: conjunctival and/or genital ulcers; rashes - typically 'target' or 'iris' lesions, or bullae on extremities; fever and malaise. No lesions on trunk.
- *Mucocutaneous lesions and systemic illness*: The major form (Stevens-Johnson syndrome) is widespread, with fever and toxicity, bullous and other rashes, pneumonia, arthritis, nephritis or myocarditis.

Incidence

Uncommon: mainly young adult males.

Aetiology

Reactions to microorganisms (herpes simplex, mycoplasma), to drugs (e.g. sulphonamides or

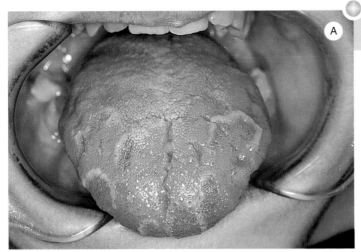

FIGURE 4.58 **Geographic tongue** (A) associated with skin psoriatic lesions (B).

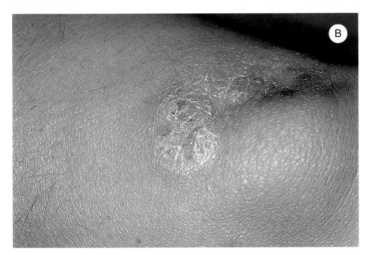

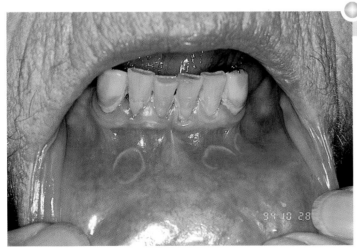

FIGURE 4.59 **Geographic stomatitis.**

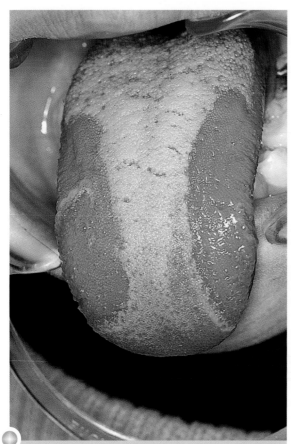

FIGURE 4.60 **Geographic tongue.**

barbiturates) or to other factors in many cases. Complement-mediated cytopathic effects may be involved.

Diagnosis

Clinical; biopsy sometimes helpful.

Differentiate from other lip lesions and other causes of mouth ulcers.

Management

- *Minor form:* symptomatic treatment.
- *Major form:* systemic corticosteroids and/or azathioprine or other immunomodulatory drugs.

References

Farthing P, Bagan JV, Scully C Mucosal disease series. Number IV. Erythema multiforme. Oral Dis 2005 Sep; 11(5):261-267

Carrozzo M, Togliatto M, Gandolfo S Erythema multiforme. A heterogeneous pathologic phenotype. Minerva Stomatol 1999 May; 48(5):217-226

Williams PM, Conklin RJ Erythema multiforme: a review and contrast from Stevens-Johnson syndrome/toxic epidermal necrolysis. Dent Clin North Am 2005 Jan; 49(1):67-76

Erythroplasia
(Erythroplakia)

Clinical features

Red velvety patch, usually level with or depressed below surrounding mucosa, commonly on soft palate or floor or mouth.

Incidence

Uncommon: mainly seen in elderly males. It is much less common than leukoplakia, but far more likely to be dysplastic or malignant.

Aetiology

See predisposing factors for carcinoma.

Diagnosis

Biopsy for epithelial dysplasia and carcinoma.

Differentiate from inflammatory and atrophic lesions, e.g. in deficiency anaemias, geographic tongue, lichen planus.

Management

Excise, but the prognosis is often poor.

References

Reichart PA, Philipsen HP Oral erythroplakia: a review. Oral Oncol 2005 Jul; 41(6):551-561

Sciubba JJ Oral precancer and cancer: etiology, clinical presentation, diagnosis, and management. Compend Contin Educ Dent 2000 Oct; 21(10A):892-898

Scully C, Felix DH Oral medicine: update for the dental practitioner: red and pigmented lesions. Br Dent J 2005 Nov 26; 199(10):639-645

Fibrous Lump or Nodule
(Fibroepithelial polyp)

Clinical features

Pedunculated or broadly sessile, sometimes ulcerated, hard or soft, mainly on buccal mucosa or elsewhere. It is termed epulis if on gingival margin.

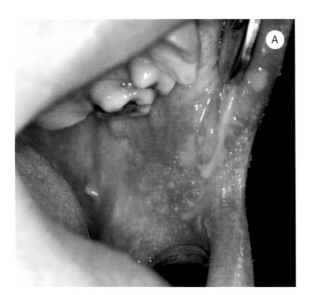

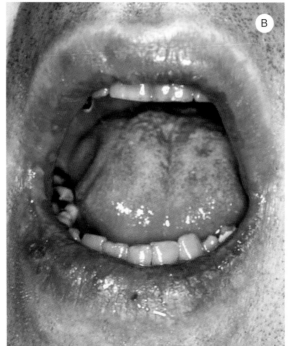

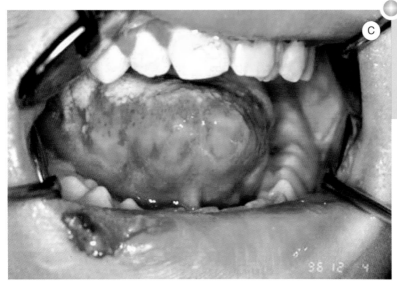

FIGURE 4.61 Erythema multiforme. The typical oral lesions are diffuse erosions mainly involving the anterior part of the mouth (A). Characteristically, the lips are involved with erosions, bleeding ulcers and crusting (B, C).

Incidence

Common.

Aetiology

Chronic irritation causing fibrous hyperplasia.

Diagnosis

Excision biopsy.

Differentiate from any other soft tissue tumour.

Management

Excise for histological confirmation.

References

Zain RB, Fei YJ Fibrous lesions of the gingiva: a histopathologic analysis of 204 cases. Oral Surg Oral Med Oral Pathol 1990 Oct; 70(4):466-470

Fissured (Scrotal) Tongue

Clinical features

Multiple fissures. Sometimes the tongue is sore. Commonly associated with erythema migrans. The condition is of no consequence.

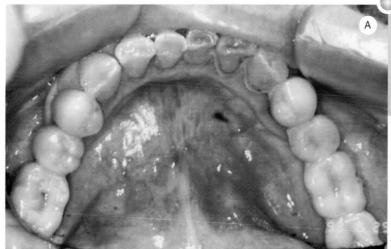

FIGURE 4.62 Oral erythroplakia
(almost all these lesions have the histological feature of in situ or micro-invasive squamous cell carcinoma). (A) Erythroplakia of the floor of the mouth. (B) Large erythroplasic lesion of the buccal mucosa.

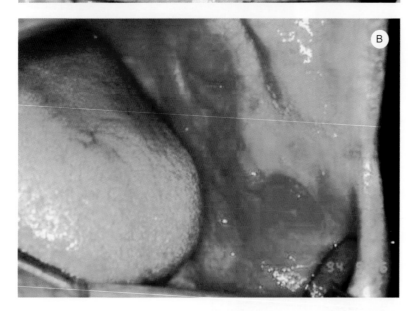

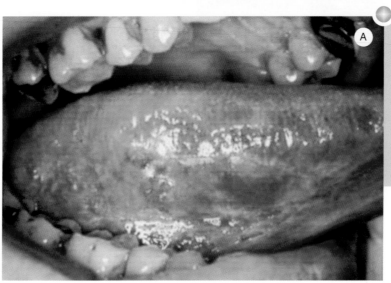

FIGURE 4.63 Oral erythroplakia.
(A) Erythroplakia of the border and the ventrum of the tongue: several areas of severe dysplasia and in situ carcinoma were found histologically. (B) Typical erythroplakia of the soft palate with histological signs of severe dysplasia. (C) Large erythroplakia involving the floor of the mouth, showing areas of moderate dysplasia and invasive carcinoma histologically.

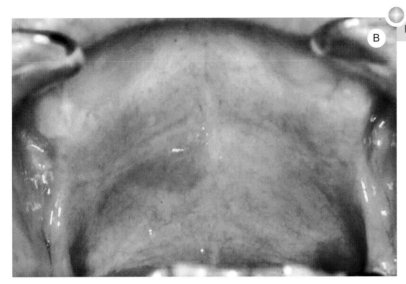

FIGURE 4.63 *Continued.*

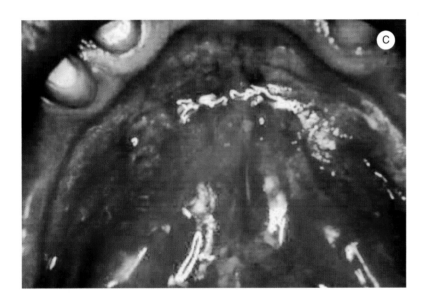

Incidence

Common (1-5%). A fissured tongue is found in normal people, often in Down syndrome and in Melkersson-Rosenthal syndrome (fissured tongue, cheilitis granulomatosa and unilateral facial nerve paralysis).

Aetiology

Often hereditary. Increases with age.

Diagnosis

None, but blood picture if tongue is sore.

The diagnosis is usually clearcut. Lobulated tongue of Sjögren's syndrome must be differentiated.

Management

Reassure.

References

Barankin B, Guenther L Dermatological manifestations of Down's syndrome. J Cutan Med Surg 2001 Jul-Aug; 5(4):289-293

Gerressen M, Ghassemi A, Stockbrink G, Riediger D, Zadeh MD Melkersson-Rosenthal syndrome: case report of a 30-year misdiagnosis. J Oral Maxillofac Surg 2005 Jul; 63(7):1035-1039

Rogers RS 3rd Melkersson-Rosenthal syndrome and orofacial granulomatosis. Dermatol Clin 1996 Apr; 14(2):371-379

Foliate Papillitis

Clinical features

Foliate papillae occasionally become inflamed or irritated, with associated enlargement and tenderness. These areas are enlarged and somewhat lobular with an intact overlying mucosa.

Incidence

Common.

Aetiology

Reactive hyperplasia of lymphoid tissue in deep crypts of foliate papillae.

Diagnosis

History and clinical features.

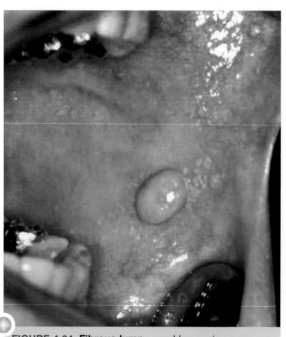

FIGURE 4.64 **Fibrous lump** caused by masticatory trauma.

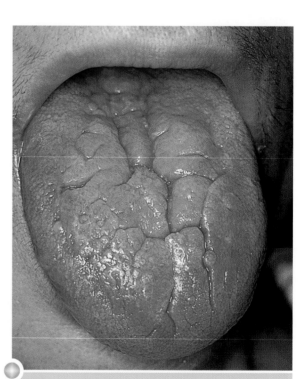

FIGURE 4.66 **Fissured (scrotal) tongue.**

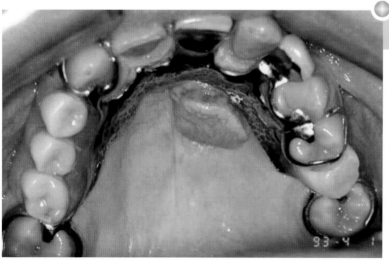

FIGURE 4.65 **Fibrous lump** caused by denture trauma.

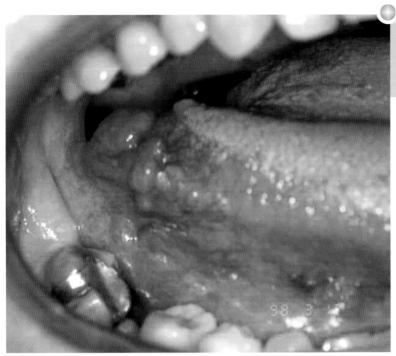

FIGURE 4.67 Foliate papillitis. These lesions have to be differentiated from the carcinoma: they are characteristically located, soft, frequently bilateral and with an intact overlying mucosa.

Differentiate from carcinoma. If carcinoma is suspected, biopsy is mandatory.

Management
Reassure.

References
Di Felice R, Lombardi T Foliate papillitis occurring in a child: a case report. Ann Dent 1993 Winter; 52(2):17-18

Fordyce's Granules

Clinical features
Multiple slightly raised whitish-yellow spots, rarely coalescing. They occur mainly in the vermilion of the upper lip, buccal mucosa and retromolar region.

Incidence
Common in adult population.

Aetiology
Development anomaly characterised by heteropic sebaceous glands in the oral mucosa.

Diagnosis
Clinical features.

Management
Reassurance. No treatment is required.

References
Daley TD Intraoral sebaceous hyperplasia. Diagnostic criteria. Oral Surg Oral Med Oral Pathol 1993 Mar; 75(3):343-347

Kaminagakura E, Andrade CR, Rangel AL, Coletta RD, Graner E, Almeida OP, Vargas PA Sebaceous adenoma of oral cavity: report of case and comparative proliferation study with sebaceous gland hyperplasia and Fordyce's granules. Oral Dis 2003 Nov; 9(6): 323-327

Nordstrom KM, McGinley KJ, Lessin SR, Leyden JJ Neutral lipid composition of Fordyce's granules. Br J Dermatol 1989 Nov, 121(5):669-670

Furred Tongue

Clinical features
The tongue has yellowish 'fur', which may be discoloured by foods or drugs. Halitosis often originates from the tongue.

Incidence
Common in febrile illnesses.

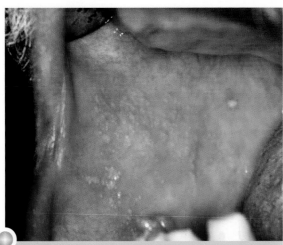

FIGURE 4.68 **Fordyce's granules.** Multiple yellow granules in the right buccal mucosa.

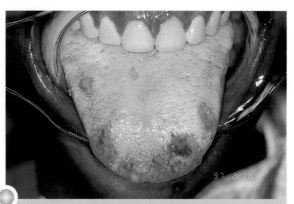

FIGURE 4.69 **Furred tongue** in a patient with erythema multiforme.

Aetiology

Often unknown, but sometimes poor oral hygiene, feverish illnesses (e.g. herpetic stomatitis), dehydration or soft diet. Debris and bacteria accumulate, especially if diet contains little roughage. An upper denture also does not clean the tongue as effectively as palatal rugae.

Diagnosis

Exclusion of the following differential diagnoses: thrush (rarely on dorsum of tongue), chronic candidosis, hairy leukoplakia (lateral borders of tongue) or other leukoplakias.

Management

Treat underlying condition.

References

Powell FC Glossodynia and other disorders of the tongue. Dermatol Clin 1987 Oct; 5(4):687-693

Glossitis Due to Candidosis

Clinical features

Diffuse erythema and soreness or rhomboidal (diamond-shaped) red, or nodular and depapillated or white, in midline of dorsum of tongue, just anterior to circumvallate papillae. There may also be patches of thrush, particularly in upper buccal sulcus posteriorly.

Incidence

Uncommon except in those with HIV infection, smokers or those taking antibiotics.

Aetiology

Opportunistic infection with candida species, particularly *C. albicans*. Predisposing factors include broad-spectrum antimicrobials (particularly tetracycline) and xerostomia, topical corticosteroids and immune defect (more often thrush).

Diagnosis

Smear for candidal hyphae.

Differentiate from deficiency glossitis.

Management

Treat predisposing cause, smoking cessation, antifungals.

References

McCullough MJ, Savage NW Oral candidosis and the therapeutic use of antifungal agents in dentistry. Aust Dent J 2005 Dec; 50(4 suppl 2):S36-39

Terai H, Shimahara M Atrophic tongue associated with Candida. J Oral Pathol Med 2005 Aug; 34(7):397-400

Glossitis in Deficiency States

Clinical features

Tongue may appear completely normal or there may be linear or patchy red lesions, depapillation with erythema, or pallor. There may also be oral ulceration and angular stomatitis.

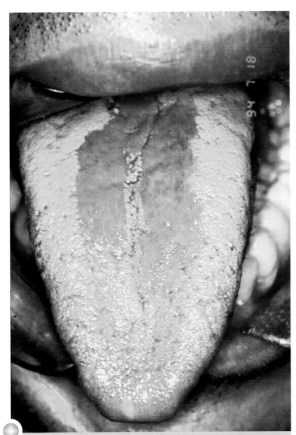

FIGURE 4.70 Candidal glossitis after prolonged antibiotic treatment.

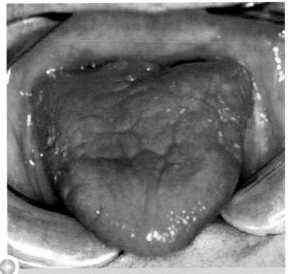

FIGURE 4.71 HIV–related **candidal glossitis.**

Incidence

Uncommon, except in malabsorption states, pernicious anaemia or the occasional vegan or other dietary preferance.

Aetiology

Deficiencies of iron, folic acid, vitamin B_{12} (rarely other B vitamins).

Diagnosis

Blood picture and vitamin assays. Biopsy rarely indicated.

Differentiate from erythema migrans, lichen planus and acute candidosis.

Management

Replacement therapy *after underlying cause of deficiency established and rectified.*

References

Carethers M Diagnosing vitamin B12 deficiency, a common geriatric disorder. Geriatrics 1988 Mar; 43(3):89-94

Field EA, Speechley JA, Rugman FR, Varga E, Tyldesley WR Oral signs and symptoms in patients with undiagnosed vitamin B12 deficiency. J Oral Pathol Med 1995 Nov; 24(10):468-470

Lu SY, Wu HC Initial diagnosis of anemia from sore mouth and improved classification of anemias by MCV and RDW in 30 patients. Oral Surg Oral Med Oral Pathol Oral Radiol Endod 2004 Dec; 98(6):679-685

Granular Cell Myoblastoma

Clinical features

The tumour is rounded or ovoid with rather indefinite margins. It is flesh-coloured to pink or yellow and is situated beneath the epithelium of the tongue. It is between 5 and 20 mm in size.

Incidence

Uncommon.

Aetiology

Unknown.

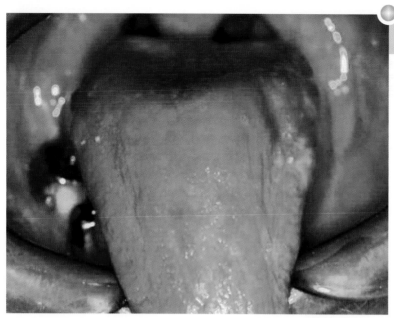

FIGURE 4.72 **Glossitis** in iron deficiency anaemia.

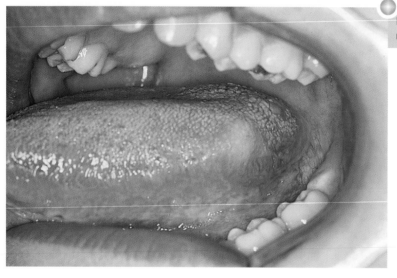

FIGURE 4.73 **Granular cell myoblastoma.**

Diagnosis

Histopathologic examination is needed for the diagnosis.

Management

Surgical excision is the only treatment.

References

Becelli R, Perugini M, Gasparini G, Cassoni A, Fabiani F Abrikossoff's tumor. J Craniofac Surg 2001 Jan; 12(1):78-81

Chrysomali E, Papanicolaou SI, Dekker NP, Regezi JA Benign neural tumors of the oral cavity: a comparative immunohistochemical study. Oral Surg Oral Med Oral Pathol Oral Radiol Endod 1997 Oct; 84(4):381-390

Haemangioma

Clinical features

Red or blue, painless, soft and sometimes fluctuant lesion that usually blanches on pressure. Most appear in infancy and are single.

Incidence

Most common on tongue, vermilion of lip or buccal mucosa.

Aetiology

Hamartoma or benign tumour. Multiple tumours are present in Maffucci's syndrome. Oral haemangiomas are present in Sturge-Weber and Von Hippel-Lindau syndromes.

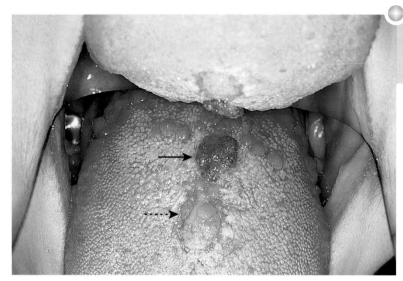

FIGURE 4.74 Haemangioma (continuous arrow) and **lymphangioma** (interrupted arrow) of the dorsum of the tongue.

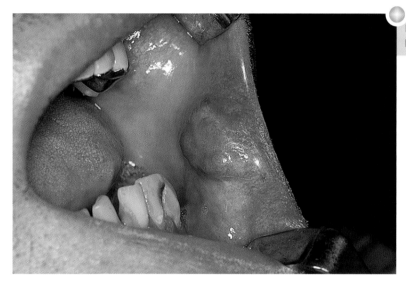

FIGURE 4.75 Cavernous haemangioma of the buccal mucosa.

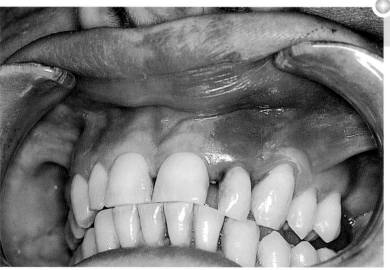

FIGURE 4.76 Flat haemangioma of the gingiva and sulcus.

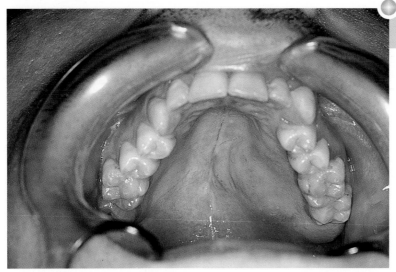

FIGURE 4.77 Cavernous haemangioma of the palate.

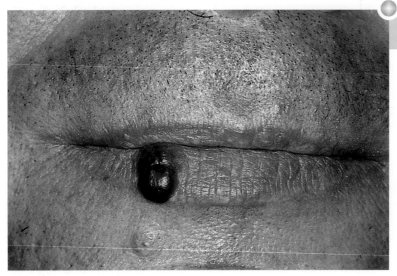

FIGURE 4.78 Haemangioma of the lower lip.

Diagnosis

Usually is clinical. *Rarely,* aspiration biopsy (excision if feasible) for confirmation.

Differentiate from telangiectasia, purpura, Kaposi's sarcoma and epithelioid angiomatosis.

Management

Observation (some 50% regress spontaneously), cryosurgery, argon laser, sclerosant or (rarely) arterial embolisation - only if bleeding is troublesome.

References

Ilgenli T, Canda T, Canda S, Unal T, Baylas H Oral giant pyogenic granulomas associated with facial skin hemangiomas (Sturge-Weber syndrome). Periodontal Clin Investig 1999; 21(2):28-32

Johann AC, Aguiar MC, do Carmo MA, Gomez RS, Castro WH, Mesquita RA Sclerotherapy of benign oral vascular lesion with ethanolamine oleate: an open clinical trial with 30 lesions. Oral Surg Oral Med Oral Pathol Oral Radiol Endod 2005 Nov; 100(5):579-584

Korf BR The phakomatoses. Clin Dermatol 2005 Jan-Feb; 23(1):78-84

Lee NH, Choi EH, Choi WK, Lee SH, Ahn SK Maffucci's syndrome with oral and intestinal haemangioma. Br J Dermatol 1999 May; 140(5):968-969

Liu DG, Ma XC, Li BM, Zhang JG Clinical study of preoperative angiography and embolization of hypervascular neoplasms in the oral and maxillofacial region. Oral Surg Oral Med Oral Pathol Oral Radiol Endod 2006 Jan; 101(1):102-109

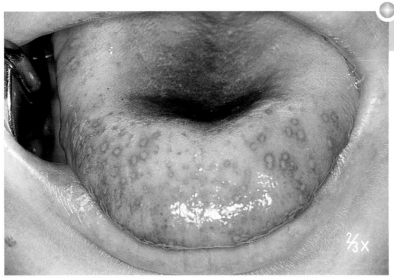

FIGURE 4.79 Hand, foot and mouth disease.

Hand, Foot and Mouth Disease

Clinical features

Incubation period is 2-6 days. Infections may be subclinical. Clinical features include: oral ulcers, resembling herpetic stomatitis but affecting labial and buccal mucosa; no gingivitis; mild fever, malaise and anorexia; rash - red papules that evolve to superficial vesicles in a few days, found mainly on the palms and soles.

Aetiology

Coxsackie viruses (usually A16; rarely A5 or 10).

Incidence

Common. It usually occurs in small epidemics, in children.

Diagnosis

Clinical. Serology is confirmatory but rarely required.

Differentiate from herpetic stomatitis and chickenpox.

Management

Symptomatic (see herpes simplex).

References

Cabral LA, Almeida JD, de Oliveira ML, Meza AC
  Hand, foot, and mouth disease: a case report.
  Quintessence Int 1998 Mar; 29(3):194-196
Frydenberg A, Starr M Hand, foot and mouth disease.
  Aust Fam Physician 2003 Aug; 32(8):594-595

Lopez-Sanchez A, Guijarro Guijarro B, Hernandez Vallejo G Human repercussions of foot and mouth disease and other similar viral diseases. Med Oral 2003 Jan-Feb; 8(1):26-32

Herpangina

Clinical features

Incubation period is 2-9 days. Many infections are subclinical. Clinical features include: pharyngeal ulcers, no gingivitis, cervical lymphadenitis (moderate), fever, malaise, irritability, anorexia and vomiting.

Incidence

Uncommon. Small outbreaks are seen among young children.

Aetiology

Coxsackie viruses (usually A7, 9, 16; B1, 2, 3, 4 or 5); ECHO viruses (9 or 17).

Diagnosis

Clinical. Serology (theoretically) is confirmatory.

Differentiate from herpetic stomatitis and chickenpox.

Management

Symptomatic (see herpes simplex).

References

Fenton SJ, Unkel JH Viral infections of the oral mucosa in children: a clinical review. Pract Periodontics Aesthet Dent 1997 Aug; 9(6):683-690

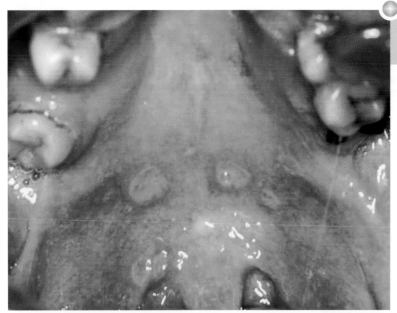

FIGURE 4.80 Herpangina. Four aphthous-like ulcerations can be seen on the soft palate.

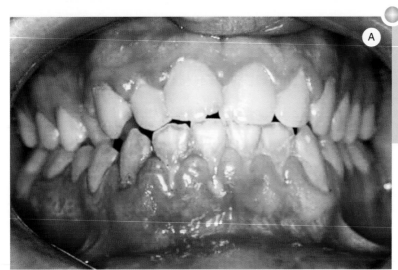

FIGURE 4.81 Herpetic gingivo-stomatitis in young adults. Note: the diffuse red appearance of the swollen gingiva (A, B); the erosions and the lip involvement (B, C). The gingival involvement is important for the differential diagnosis from erythema multiforme.

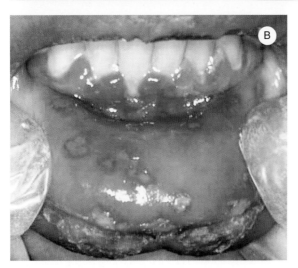

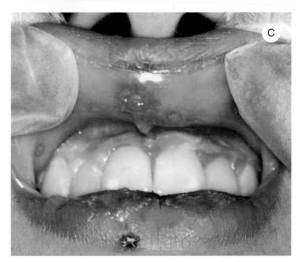

Zavate O, Avram G, Pavlov E, Burlea-Iriciuc A, Ivan A, Cotor F Coxsackie A virus-associated herpetiform angina. Virologie 1984 Jan-Mar, 35(1):49-53

Herpes Simplex Infections
Herpetic stomatitis

Clinical features

Incubation period is 3-7 days.

Mouth ulcers: multiple vesicles and round scattered ulcers with yellow slough and erythematous halo; ulcers fuse to produce irregular lesions.

Gingivitis: diffuse erythema and oedema, occasionally haemorrhagic.

Cervical lymphadenitis.

Fever.

Malaise, irritability and *anorexia.*

Incidence

Common cause of mouth ulcers in poor areas, with fever in children. It is also seen in adults, especially in more affluent communities.

Aetiology

Herpes simplex virus (HSV), usually type 1.

Diagnosis

Differentiate from other causes of mouth ulcers, especially hand, foot and mouth disease, chickenpox and shingles, herpangina, erythema multiforme and leukaemia. Smear for viral-damaged cells or immunostaining. Viral culture or electron microscopy is used occasionally. A rising titre of antibodies is confirmatory.

Management

Soft diet and adequate fluid intake, antipyretics/analgesics (paracetamol/acetaminophen elixir), local antiseptics (0.2% aqueous chlorhexidine mouthwashes), aciclovir orally or parenterally in immunocompromised patients.

Herpes labialis

Clinical features

Prodromal paraesthesia or irritation. Erythema, then vesicles at/near mucocutaneous junction of lip. Heals in 7-10 days.

Incidence

Common, especially in immunocompromised.

Aetiology

Herpes simplex virus (HSV), usually type 1. HSV latent in trigeminal ganglion is reactivated by sun, trauma, menstruation, fever, HIV disease, immunosuppression, etc.

Diagnosis

Viral damage can be confirmed by smear.

Differentiate from zoster, impetigo or (rarely) carcinoma.

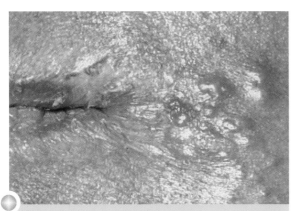

FIGURE 4.82 Recurrent herpes labialis with cutaneous involvement.

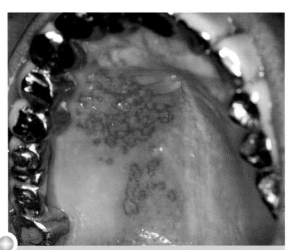

FIGURE 4.83 Recurrent intraoral herpes. On the unilateral right hard palate several little erosions that coalesce may be seen.

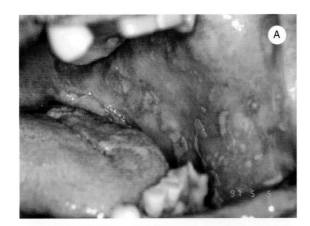

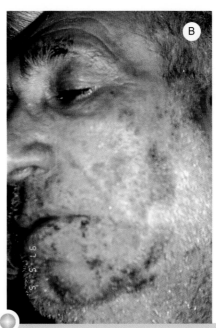

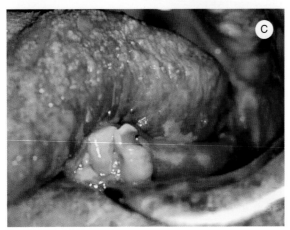

FIGURE 4.84 Herpes zoster: typical unilateral mucosal and skin erosive lesions from involvement of the second and third trigeminal branches (A, B, C). On the skin, crusts are also evident (B).

Management

Penciclovir 1% cream or aciclovir 5% cream applied in prodrome. Immunocompromised may need systemic aciclovir (oral or i.v.).

Recurrent intra-oral herpes

Clinical features

Localised area of unilateral vesiculation followed by ulceration (erosion).

Incidence

Rare.

Diagnosis

Viral damage can be confirmed by smear.

Differentiate from zoster or herpetiform ulcers (recurrent herpes is monolateral).

Management

Aciclovir: 5% cream applied in prodrome. Immunocompromised patients may need systemic aciclovir (oral or i.v.), famciclovir or valaciclovir.

Herpes Varicella-Zoster Virus Infections
Chickenpox (varicella)

Clinical features

Incubation period is 14-21 days.

Ulcers: indistinguishable from HSV, but no associated gingivitis.

Rash: mainly face and trunk; papules then vesicles, pustules and scabs, in crops.

Cervical lymphadenitis.

Fever.

Malaise, irritability, anorexia.

Incidence
Common childhood exanthem.

Aetiology
Herpes varicella-zoster virus (VZV).

Diagnosis
Clinical. Immunostained smear or rising antibody titre are confirmatory.

Differentiate from other mouth ulcers, especially herpes simplex and other viral infections.

Management
Symptomatic; immune globulin or aciclovir or famciclovir or valaciclovir in immunocompromised.

Shingles (Zoster)

Clinical features
Pain: before, with and after rash.

Rash: unilateral vesiculating then scabbing in dermatome. Majority thoracic: 30% trigeminal region.

Mouth ulcers: *mandibular zoster* - ipsilateral on buccal and lingual mucosa; *maxillary* - ipsilateral on palate and vestibule.

Incidence
Uncommon. Mainly affects elderly, or immunocompromised, such as in HIV infection or cancer.

Aetiology
Reactivation of VZV latent in sensory ganglia. Immune defects predispose to reactivation.

Diagnosis
Clinical. Differentiate from toothache and other causes of ulcers, especially herpes simplex.

Management
Analgesics; aciclovir, famciclovir or valaciclovir (high dose) orally or parenterally, especially in the immunocompromised; symptomatic treatment of ulcers.

Ophthalmic zoster: ophthalmological opinion.

References
Huber MA Herpes simplex type-1 virus infection. Quintessence Int 2003 Jun; 34(6):453-467

McCullough MJ, Savage NW Oral viral infections and the therapeutic use of antiviral agents in dentistry. Aust Dent J 2005 Dec; 50(4 Suppl 2):S31-S35

Nikkels AF, Pierard GE Oral antivirals revisited in the treatment of herpes zoster: what do they accomplish? Am J Clin Dermatol 2002; 3(9):591-598

Siegel MA Diagnosis and management of recurrent herpes simplex infections. J Am Dent Assoc 2002 Sep; 133(9):1245-1249

Stoopler ET Oral herpetic infections (HSV 1-8). Dent Clin North Am 2005 Jan; 49(1):15-29

Stoopler ET, Pinto A, DeRossi SS, Sollecito TP Herpes simplex and varicella-zoster infections: clinical and laboratory diagnosis. Gen Dent 2003 May-Jun; 51(3):281-286

Human Immunodeficiency Virus Disease

Clinical features
Oral lesions in HIV disease have been classified as follows:

Group I *Lesions strongly associated with HIV infection*:

- Candidosis
  Erythematous
  Hyperplastic
  Thrush
- Hairy leukoplakia (EBV)
- HIV-gingivitis
- Necrotising ulcerative gingivitis
- HIV-periodontitis

- Kaposi's sarcoma
- Non-Hodgkin's lymphoma.

Group II *Lesions less commonly associated with HIV infection:*

- Atypical ulceration (oropharyngeal)
- Idopathic thrombocytopenic purpura
- Salivary gland diseases
  Dry mouth
  Unilateral or bilateral swelling of major salivary glands
- Viral infections (other than EBV)
  Cytomegalovirus
  Herpes simplex virus
  Human papillomavirus (warty-like lesions): condyloma acuminatum, focal epithelial hyperplasia and verruca vulgaris
  Varicella-zoster virus: herpes zoster and varicella.

Group III *Lesions possibly associated with HIV infection:*

- A miscellany of rare diseases.

References

Eyeson JD, Warnakulasuriya KA, Johnson NW Prevalence and incidence of oral lesions: the changing scene. Oral Dis 2000 Sep; 6(5):267-273

Patton LL, Phelan JA, Ramos-Gomez FJ, Nittayananta W, Shiboski CH, Mbuguye TL Prevalence and classification of HIV-associated oral lesions. Oral Dis 2002; 8 Suppl 2:98-2:109

Ryder MI Periodontal management of HIV-infected patients. Periodontol 2000 2000 Jun; 23:85-93

Infectious Mononucleosis

Clinical features

Incubation period is probably 15-21 days.

Sore throat, faucial swelling and ulceration with creamy exudate and palatal petechiae; occasional mouth ulcers; lymph node enlargement - generalised tender lymphadenopathy; fever, malaise, anorexia and lassitude.

Incidence

Common: predominantly a disease of adolescents.

Aetiology

Epstein-Barr virus (EBV).

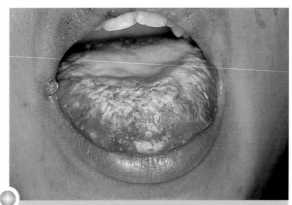

FIGURE 4.85 Mononucleosis. Vesiculo-erosive lesions.

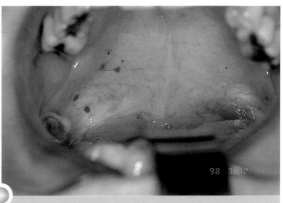

FIGURE 4.86 Mononucleosis. Palatal petechiae.

Diagnosis

Clinical, confirmed by blood picture and Paul-Bunnell test for heterophil antibodies.

Differentiate from other glandular fever-like syndromes, especially early HIV infection, cytomegalovirus infection, *Toxoplasma gondii* infection and diphtheria.

Management

Symptomatic (see herpes simplex); metronidazole may improve sore throat.

References

Ebell MH Epstein-Barr virus infectious mononucleosis. Am Fam Physician 2004 Oct 1; 70(7):1279-1287

Kawa K Epstein-Barr virus-associated diseases in humans. Int J Hematol 2000 Feb; 71(2):108-117

Kaposi's Sarcoma

Clinical features

Early lesions are red, purple or brown macules. Long-standing lesions tend to be blue or black nodular and may ulcerate, extend, or disseminate. Kaposi's sarcoma typically involves the palate, but can affect any other oral site.

Incidence

Once rare, now seen in HIV infection.

Aetiology

Unclear: a malignant neoplasm of endothelial cells. It is frequently associated with HIV infection and may be due to human herpesvirus 8. Seen mainly in AIDS or immunosuppressed organ transplant patients

Diagnosis

Biopsy is confirmatory.

Differentiate from other pigmented lesions, especially epithelioid angiomatosis, haemangiomas and purpura.

Management

Treatment of underlying predisposing condition if possible; vinca alkaloids systemically or intralesionally; radiotherapy.

References

Antman K, Chang Y Kaposi's sarcoma. N Engl J Med 2000 Apr 6; 342(14):1027-1038

Epstein JB, Cabay RJ, Glick M Oral malignancies in HIV disease: changes in disease presentation, increasing understanding of molecular pathogenesis, and current management. Oral Surg Oral Med Oral Pathol Oral Radiol Endod 2005 Nov; 100(5):571-578

Leao JC, Porter S, Scully C Human herpesvirus 8 and oral health care: an update. Oral Surg Oral Med Oral Pathol Oral Radiol Endod 2000 Dec; 90(6):694-704

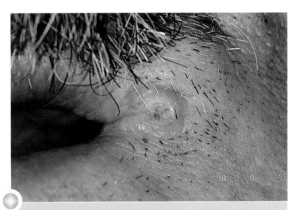

FIGURE 4.88 **Keratoacanthoma.** A painless ulcer-like crater is evident close to the commissural area.

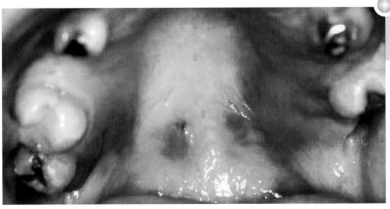

FIGURE 4.87 **Kaposi's sarcoma** of the palate. HIV-positive patient having early red-purple macules.

Wood C, Harrington W Jr AIDS and associated malignancies. Cell Res 2005 Nov-Dec; 15(11-12): 947-952

Keratoacanthoma

Clinical features

This a cutaneous benign lesion that occurs almost exclusively on the lips, typically on the vermilion border.

Characteristically, the keratoacanthoma has raised margins around a central ulcer-like crater filled with keratin. Very rarely, intra-oral keratoacanthoma has been reported.

Incidence

Rare.

Aetiology

Unknown.

Diagnosis

Biopsy is confirmatory.

Differentiate from carcinoma.

Management

Surgical excision is the only treatment.

References

Chen YK, Lin LM, Lin CC, Chen CH
Keratoacanthoma of the tongue: a diagnostic problem. Otolaryngol Head Neck Surg 2003 Apr; 128(4):581-582

Habel G, O'Regan B, Eissing A, Khoury F, Donath K Intra-oral keratoacanthoma: an eruptive variant and review of the literature. Br Dent J 1991 May 11; 170(9):336-339

Schwartz RA Keratoacanthoma. J Am Acad Dermatol 1994 Jan; 30(1):1-19

Keratoses

Oral white plaques characterised by increased keratinisation are called keratoses. When an aetiologic factor is found (e.g. trauma from teeth) they are classified according to the aetiology. Leukoplakia is the term used for hyperkeratotic white mucosal lesions that cannot be classified in another way. Leukoplakia is either of unknown cause or caused by smoking. There are no specific histopathological connotations.

Most keratoses are benign. Overall, 1-3% are premalignant. Keratoses in particular sites or of particular appearance tend to have higher premalignant potential, but epithelial dysplasia, microscopically, is a more reliable guide.

Clinical features

Leukoplakia

There are three main types of leukoplakia: most are smooth plaques (homogeneous leukoplakias), some warty (verrucous leukoplakia) and some mixed white and red lesions (speckled leukoplakias). In general, homogeneous leukoplakias are benign. Premalignant potential is higher in verrucous leukoplakias, and is highest in speckled leukoplakias. Some studies show

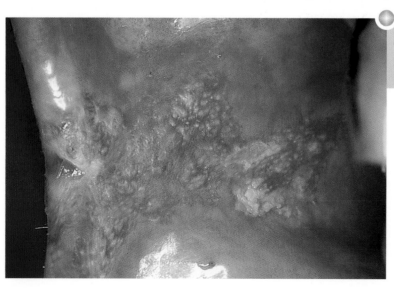

FIGURE 4.89 Candidal leukoplakia. The clinical appearance is that of non-homogeneous leukoplakia. The diagnosis is made by histological examination.

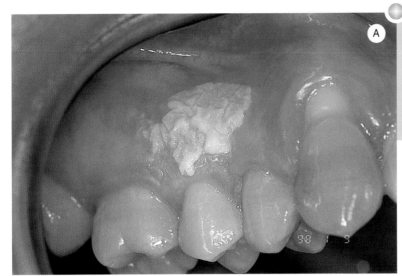

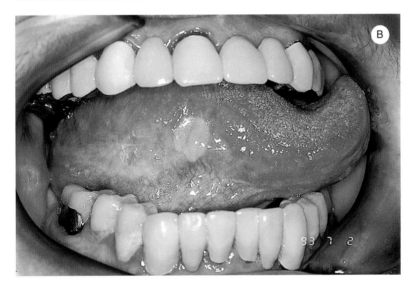

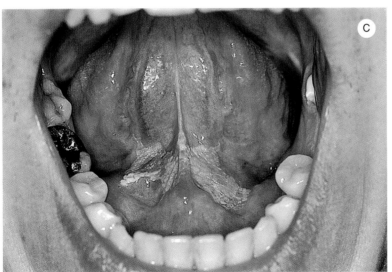

FIGURE 4.90 Leukoplakia.
(A) Homogeneous gingival leukoplakia with slight verrucous appearance.
(B) Typical appearance of homogenous leukoplakia on the border of the tongue.
(C) Non-homogeneous leukoplakia of the floor of the mouth with verrucous and erythematous areas.

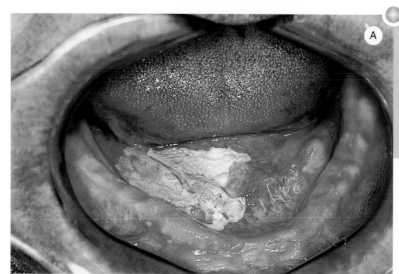

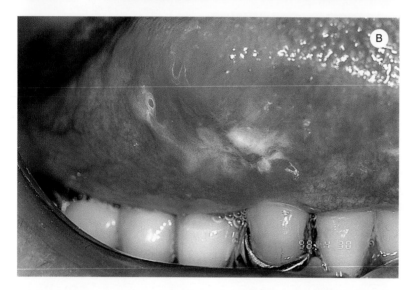

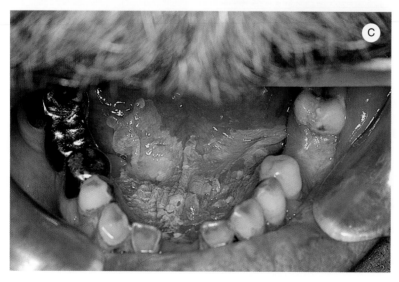

FIGURE 4.91 Leukoplakia. (A) Non-homogeneous leukoplakia of the floor of the mouth with erythematous and ulcerative features. (B) Non-homogeneous leukoplakia of the border of the tongue with an intense erythematous area. (C) Non-homogeneous verrucous leukoplakia of the floor of the mouth.

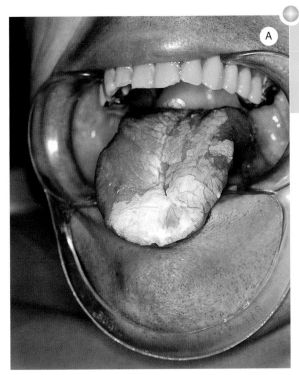

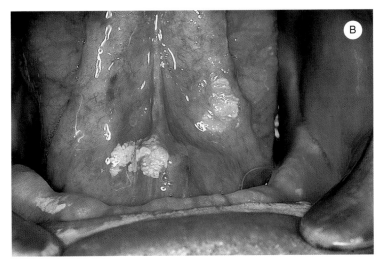

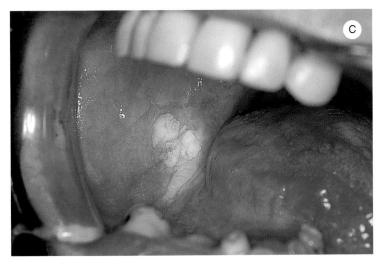

FIGURE 4.92 Leukoplakia.
(A) Lingual leukoplakia in a tobacco-chewer (tobacco-associated keratosis). (B) Non-homogeneous leukoplakia of the ventrum of the tongue and of the floor of the mouth. Note the multiple white patches and the red area. (C) Verrucous leukoplakia of the buccal mucosa.

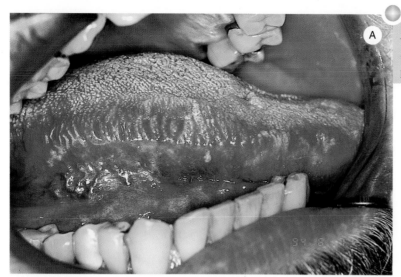

A

FIGURE 4.93 Hairy leukoplakia.
Vertical white striae on the borders of
the tongue (A, B) in a HIV-positive
patient.

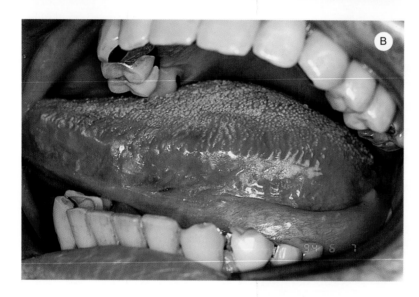

malignant transformation in over 20% of speckled
leukoplakias. The most common sites are buccal
mucosa, floor of the mouth, retrocommissural
areas, border and sulcus of the tongue.

Candidal leukoplakia
C. albicans can cause
or colonise other keratoses, particularly in
smokers, and is especially likely to form speckled
leukoplakias at commissures. It may be dysplastic
and have higher premalignant potential than some
other keratoses. Candidal leukoplakias may
respond to antifungals and stopping smoking.

Syphilitic leukoplakia
Leukoplakia,
especially of the dorsum of tongue, is a feature of
tertiary syphilis but is rarely seen now.
Premalignant potential is high.

Hairy leukoplakia
Usually has a corrugated
surface and affects margins of the tongue almost
exclusively. It is seen in the immunocompromised
and is a complication of HIV infection. It is seen
in all groups at risk of HIV infection. The
condition appears to be benign, and self-limiting.

Leukoplakia in chronic renal failure
Symmetrical soft keratosis may complicate chronic
renal failure, but resolves after treatment by renal
transplantation or dialysis.

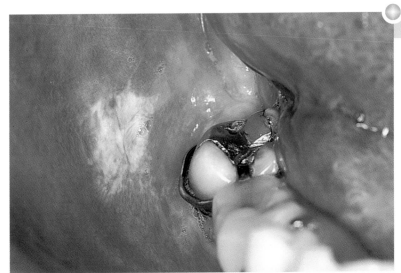

FIGURE 4.94 Frictional keratosis.

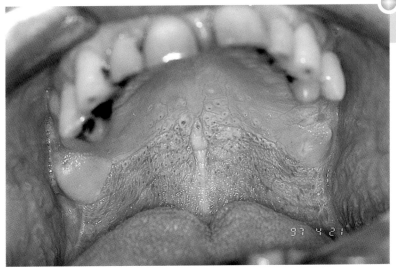

FIGURE 4.95 Smoker's keratosis.
This patient was a pipe smoker.

Frictional keratosis

Usually seen at sites of trauma from teeth, also along buccal occlusal line and occasionally beside an outstanding tooth, or on edentulous ridge. It is homogeneous and clears when irritation is removed.

Smoker's keratosis
('Stomatitis nicotina')

Pipe smoking is the usual cause. The palate, particularly the soft palate, is affected. Red orifices of swollen minor salivary glands of the palate within a widespread white lesion give a striking appearance of red spots on a white background. The lesion is benign in itself, but carcinoma may develop nearby.

Other tobacco-related habits

Tobacco chewing, snuff dipping or chewing of betel quids may lead to keratoses, which can be premalignant. Snuff dipping is associated predominantly with verrucous keratoses, which can progress to verrucous carcinoma. Tobacco-related keratoses typically resolve on stopping the habit.

Sublingual keratosis

Keratoses in the floor of the mouth/ventrum of tongue were formerly thought to be naevi (congenital) but, although of unknown aetiology, are now reported to undergo premalignant transformation. Often homogeneous, there may

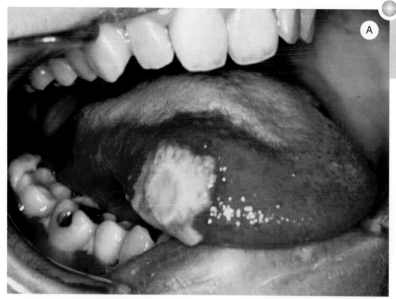

FIGURE 4.96 Acute leukaemia.
Lingual (A) and gingival (B) ulcers in a young female with acute myelomonocytic leukaemia.

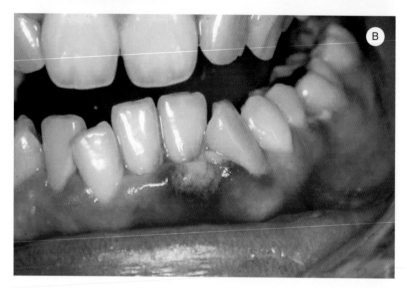

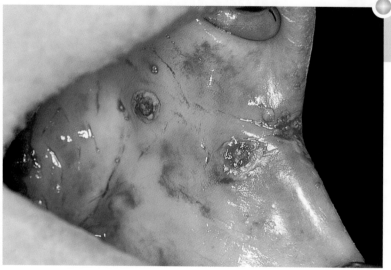

FIGURE 4.97 Acute leukaemia. Left buccal mucosal petechiae and necrotic ulcers in a patient with acute leukaemia.

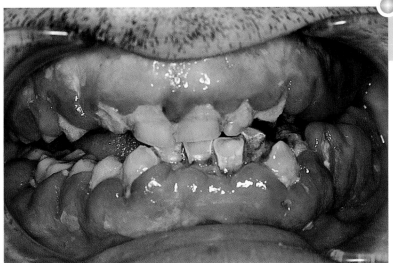

FIGURE 4.98 Acute leukaemia. Generalised gingival swelling in a patient with acute myeloblastic leukaemia.

be speckled areas. The surface has an 'ebbing tide' appearance.

Incidence

Fairly common. Keratoses are seen mainly in middle-aged/elderly adults, but hairy leukoplakia is seen mainly in young adult males.

Aetiology

Idiopathic: most cases

Friction

Tobacco: pipe smoking can cause 'nicotinic stomatitis' of the palate especially; smokeless tobacco or betel chewing can cause keratosis, usually of the buccal sulcus.

Microorganisms:
- *Candida albicans.* Candidal leukoplakias frequently appear speckled, often affect commissures and have a fairly high premalignant potential.
- *Syphilis.* Syphilitic leukoplakia especially affects dorsum of tongue and has a high premalignant potential.
- *'Hairy' leukoplakia* is virtually pathognomonic of HIV infection. Epstein-Barr virus may be detected. It is not premalignant.
- *Focal epithelial hyperplasia* (Heck's disease) is rare. It predominantly affects Inuits and Native Americans and is caused by human papillomavirus (HPV).

Diagnosis

Most white lesions need to be biopsied for possible dysplasia or early malignant change.

Differentiate from other oral white lesions.

Management

Opinions vary, but in general:
- treat predisposing factors
- surgically remove small discrete lesions <2 cm diameter and any with moderate or severe dysplasia
- observe regularly larger lesions
- consider use of retinoids.

References

Lodi G, Sardella A, Bez C, Demarosi F, Carrassi A Interventions for treating oral leukoplakia. Cochrane Database Syst Rev 2004; (3):CD001829

Petti S Pooled estimate of world leukoplakia prevalence: a systematic review. Oral Oncol 2003 Dec; 39(8): 770-780

Scully C, Porter S ABC of oral health. Swellings and red, white, and pigmented lesions. BMJ 2000 Jul 22; 321(7255):225-228

Scully C, Porter SR Orofacial disease: update for the dental clinical team: 3. White lesions. Dent Update 1999 Apr; 26(3):123-129

Sitheeque MA, Samaranayake LP Chronic hyper-plastic candidosis/candidiasis (candidal leukoplakia). Crit Rev Oral Biol Med 2003; 14(4):253-267

van der Waal I, Axell T Oral leukoplakia: a proposal for uniform reporting. Oral Oncol 2002 Sep; 38(6):521-526

Carcinoma

Keratinising carcinomas may appear as oral white lesions *ab initio* or may occasionally arise in other oral white lesions, notably in some keratoses, dyskeratosis congenita, oral submucous fibrosis or lichen planus.

Leukaemia

Clinical features

Generalised lymph node enlargement; pallor; hepatosplenomegaly; purpura; oral ulcers; cervical lymph node enlargement; petechiae and gingival haemorrhage; infections - candidosis or herpetic; others - gingival swelling (acute myeloid leukaemia), labial anaesthesia and facial palsy (rarely).

Incidence

Uncommon.

Aetiology

Idiopathic, irradiation, some chromosomal disorders, chemicals, viruses.

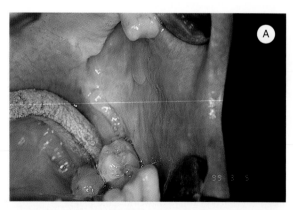

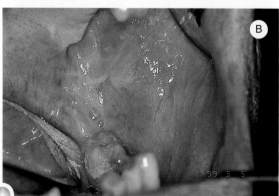

FIGURE 4.99 **Leukoedema** of the buccal mucosa (A) dissipating after stretching (B).

Diagnosis

Full blood picture and bone marrow biopsy.

Differentiate from other causes of mouth ulcers and lymph node enlargement.

Management

Chemotherapy for leukaemia; supportive care - oral hygiene and topical analgesics; aciclovir for herpetic infections; antifungals for candidosis.

References

Albuquerque MA, Migliari DA, Sugaya NN, Kuroishi M, Capuano AC, Sousa SO, Cavalcanti MG Adult T-cell leukemia/lymphoma with predominant bone involvement, initially diagosed by its oral manifestation: a case report. Oral Surg Oral Med Oral Pathol Oral Radiol Endod 2005 Sep; 100(3):315-320

Amin KS, Ehsan A, McGuff HS, Albright SC Minimally differentiated acute myelogenous leukemia (AML-MO) granulocytic sarcoma presenting in the oral cavity. Oral Oncol 2002 Jul; 38(5):516-519

Porter SR, Matthews RW, Scully C Chronic lymphocytic leukaemia with gingival and palatal deposits. J Clin Periodontol 1994 Sep; 21(8):559-561

Leukoedema

Incidence

Common.

Aetiology

No definitive cause has been established.

Clinical features

Grey-white, diffuse, filmy or milky surface, is symmetrical in distribution and occurs on the buccal mucosae.

Diagnosis

With stretching of the buccal mucosae, the opaque change will dissipate.

Management

No treatment is necessary.

References

Canaan TJ, Meehan SC Variations of structure and appearance of the oral mucosa. Dent Clin North Am 2005 Jan; 49(1):1-14

Martin JL Leukoedema: a review of the literature. J Natl Med Assoc 1992 Nov; 84(11):938-940

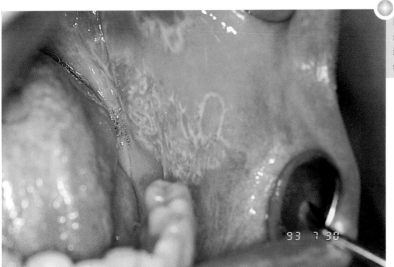

FIGURE 4.100 Oral lichen planus, reticular variety. Characteristic white interlacing keratotic striae (Wickham's striae) of the left buccal mucosa.

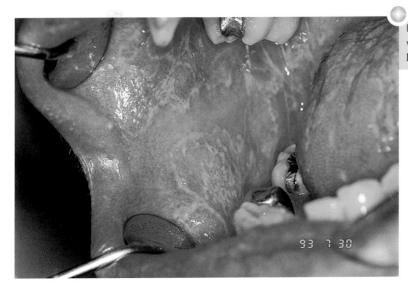

FIGURE 4.101 Oral lichen planus with papular and reticular lesions. The keratotic lines are created by papules.

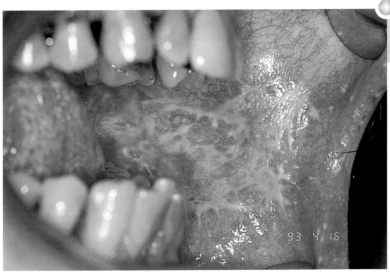

FIGURE 4.102 Oral lichen planus with usually symptomless reticular and plaque-type lesions.

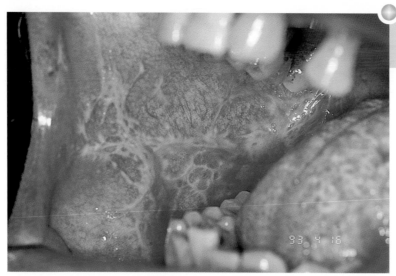

FIGURE 4.103 Oral lichen planus with papular, reticular and atrophic lesions.

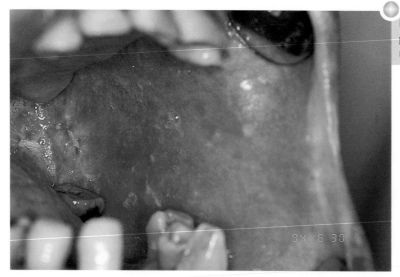

FIGURE 4.104 Oral lichen planus, predominantly atrophic. This variety may mimic erythroplakia.

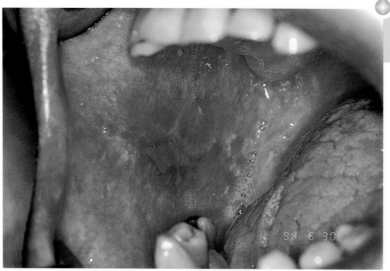

FIGURE 4.105 Oral lichen planus, atrophic variety. Note the reticular pattern surrounding the atrophic area.

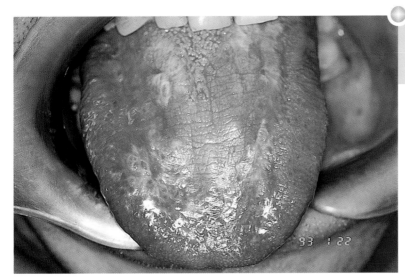

FIGURE 4.106 Oral lichen planus.
Frequently, lingual lesions have a plaque-type appearance and atrophy of the tongue papillae may be seen.

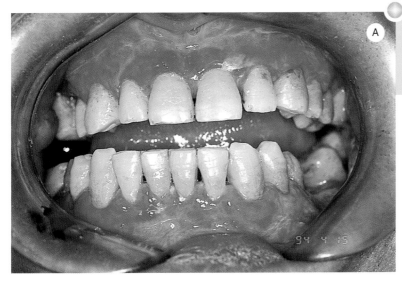

A

FIGURE 4.107 Oral lichen planus.
Gingival lesions commonly have the features of desquamative gingivitis (A). However, characteristic white reticular lesions can also be seen (B, C).

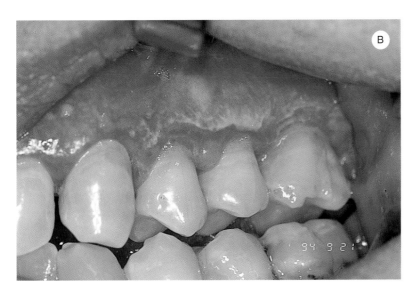

B

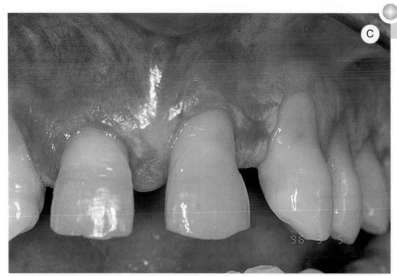

FIGURE 4.107 *Continued*.

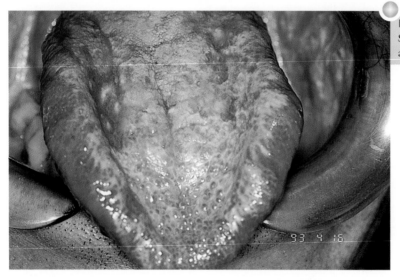

FIGURE 4.108 Oral lichen planus.
Sometimes, the classical white striae may appear on the dorsum of the tongue.

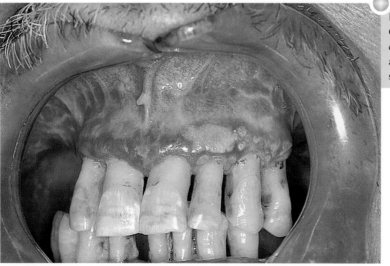

FIGURE 4.109 Oral lichen planus.
Gingival lesions of lichen planus in a cirrhotic HCV-positive patient. Red areas, white plaques and striae (in the sulcus) are visible.

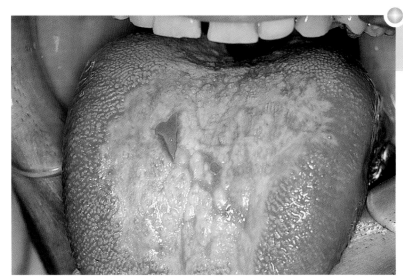

FIGURE 4.110 Oral lichen planus.
A lingual erosion surrounded by white plaques.

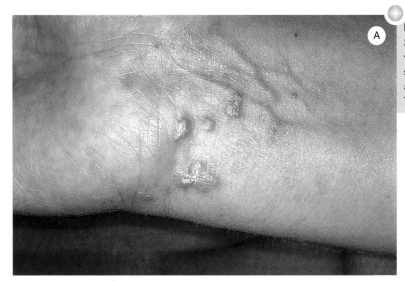

FIGURE 4.111 Oral lichen planus.
Skin lesions: small violaceous papules with mild white striae on the flexor surface of the wrists of a patient also affected by oral lichen planus (A, B). These lesions are commonly itchy.

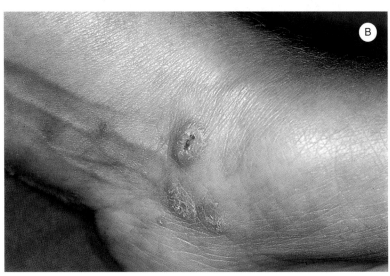

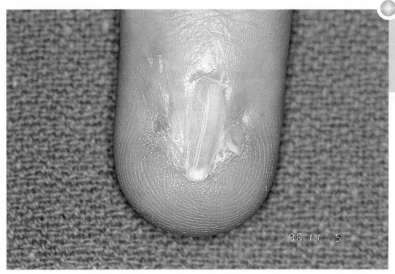

FIGURE 4.112 Oral lichen planus. Nail lesions in a patient with oral and cutaneous lichen planus. Note the onycholysis and the longitudinal striation.

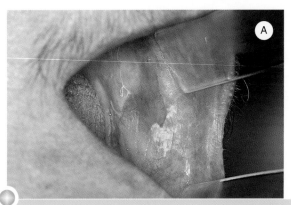
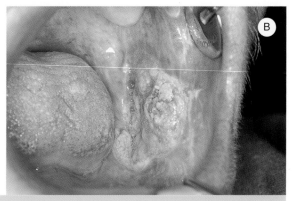

FIGURE 4.113 Oral lichen planus. Plaque-type, atrophic and reticular lesions of the left buccal mucosa in a 45-year-old woman (A). After 10 years, onset of a squamous cell carcinoma in the same buccal mucosal area (B).

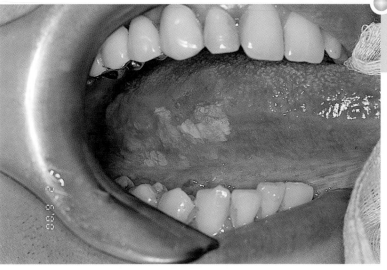

FIGURE 4.114 Oral lichen planus. A plaque-type squamous cell carcinoma in a 56-year-old woman affected for 5 years by lichen planus.

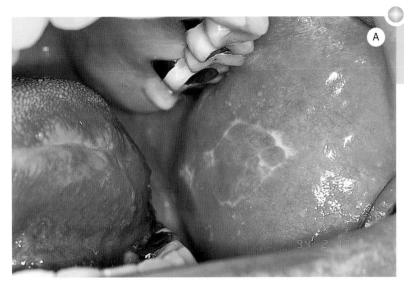

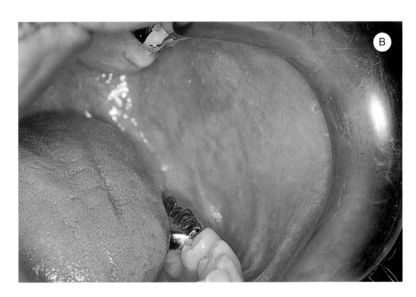

FIGURE 4.115 Oral lichen planus. Lichenoid lesions of the buccal mucosa (A) and their disappearance after substitution of the amalgam restoration (B).

Lichen Planus

Clinical features

Oral lesions tend to be bilateral, mainly in the buccal mucosae. White lesions are common; erosions are less common. There may be lesions of genital mucosa, skin or skin appendages.

Reticular lesions are most often found on the buccal mucosae, sometimes on the tongue. Papular lesions affect similar sites. Plaque-like lesions usually affect the posterior buccal mucosa. Red lesions of atrophic lichen planus (LP) may simulate erythroplasia.

Lesions may be asymptomatic or cause soreness. Erosions are irregular, persistent and painful, with a yellowish slough, and are often associated with white lesions. LP can cause 'desquamative gingivitis'.

Lichen planus can have a small premalignant potential (1% ± after 10 years).

The rash is pruritic, polygonal, purplish and papular, predominantly on flexor surfaces of wrists, and shins. Trauma may induce lesions (Koebner phenomenon).

Alopecia or nail deformities are seen occasionally. Genital lesions are typically white or erosive.

Incidence

Common: mainly middle-aged or elderly females.

Aetiology

A T-lymphocyte-mediated disorder. Usually no aetiological factor is identifiable. A minority are due to drugs, such as non-steroidal antiinflammatory drugs (lichenoid lesions), graft-versus-host disease, liver disorders, hepatitis C (possibly) and reactions to amalgam or gold (possibly).

Diagnosis

Clinical: drug history; biopsy.

Differentiate from other causes of white lesions and ulcers, especially discoid lupus erythematosus and keratoses. The 'desquamative gingivitis' of lichen planus must be differentiated from that of mucous membrane pemphigoid.

Management

Asymptomatic: no treatment; reassurance and periodical (1 to 2 times/year) examinations.

Symptomatic: corticosteroids topically and, rarely, intralesionally or systemically. Other drugs, such as retinoids or ciclosporin, have not proved reliably better or may have adverse effects. Tacrolimus may be beneficial.

References

Carrozzo M, Gandolfo S. Oral diseases possibly associated with hepatitis C virus. Crit Rev Oral Biol Med 2003; 14(2):115-127

Conrotto D, Carbone M, Carrozzo M, Arduino P, Broccoletti R, Pentenero M, Gandolfo S Ciclosporin vs. clobetasol in the topical management of atrophic and erosive oral lichen planus: a double-blind, randomized controlled trial. Br J Dermatol 2006 Jan; 154(1):139-145

Eisen D, Carrozzo M, Bagan Sebastian JV, Thongprasom K Number V Oral lichen planus: clinical features and management. Oral Dis 2005 Nov; 11(6):338-349

Gandolfo S, Richiardi L, Carrozzo M, Broccoletti R, Carbone M, Pagano M, Vestita C, Rosso S, Merletti F Risk of oral squamous cell carcinoma in 402 patients with oral lichen planus: a follow-up study in an Italian population. Oral Oncol 2004 Jan; 40(1):77-83

Lupus Erythematosus

Connective tissue disease comprising three subsets (according to the clinical gravity): systemic lupus erythematosus (SLE), subacute cutaneous (SCLE) and discoid lupus erythematosus (DLE). Oral lesions can precede other manifestations in some patients.

Clinical feature

DLE: Lesions frequently involve the skin of the face (butterfly-malar rash) and the scalp. Oral mucosa is involved in 15 to 25% of cases. The buccal mucosa, the vermilion and the gingiva are usually affected. The typical oral lesions are characterised by central erythema, white spots or papules, radiating white striae at margins and peripheral telangiectasia.

SCLE: Oral lesions look like those seen in DLE. Mild systemic symptoms are present (musculoskeletal complaints and some autoantibodies).

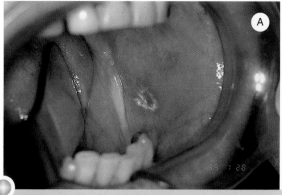 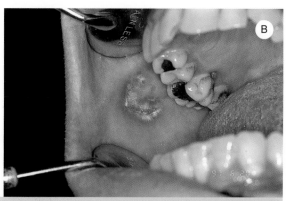

FIGURE 4.116 Lupus erythematosus. Orally, lupus lesions are characterised by erythematous areas surrounded by radiated white lines (A, B).

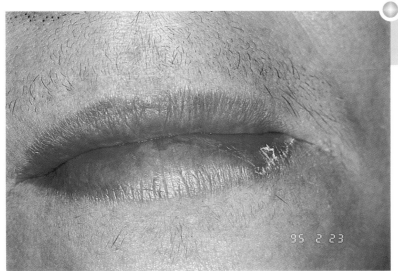

FIGURE 4.117 Lupus erythematosus. Labial lesions of discoid lupus erythematosus.

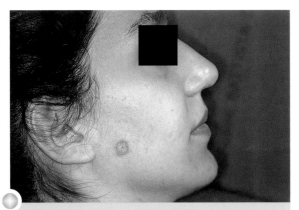

FIGURE 4.118 Lupus erythematosus. Discoid red cutaneous lesion of the cheek.

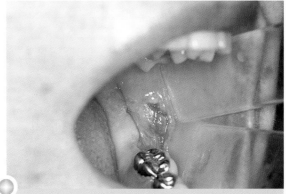

FIGURE 4.119 Lupus erythematosus. The presence of oral ulceration is one of the criteria used to diagnose systemic lupus erythematosus.

SLE: Multiple system involvement is present. Oral lesions are similar to those seen in DLE but usually with more severe ulceration. Palate is frequently involved.

Incidence
Uncommon.

Aetiology
LE is caused by an autoimmune process (involving both the humoral and the cell-mediated arms of the immune system) possibly influenced by genetic or viral factors.

Diagnosis
Biopsy (sometimes with immunostaining showing granular-linear basement membrane deposits of Ig and complement); blood test for autoantibodies: ANA and LE cell.

Differentiate from other causes of white lesions and ulcers, especially lichen planus.

Management
DLE is generally treated with topical corticosteroids. In refractory cases antimalarials or sulfones should be used. In SLE, systemic steroids and other immunosuppressive agents are used. Patients with SLE are usually followed up in rheumatological units.

References
Brennan MT, Valerin MA, Napenas JJ, Lockhart PB
  Oral manifestations of patients with lupus

erythematosus. Dent Clin North Am 2005 Jan; 49(1):127-141

Orteu CH, Buchanan JA, Hutchison I, Leigh IM, Bull RH Systemic lupus erythematosus presenting with oral mucosal lesions: easily missed? Br J Dermatol 2001 Jun; 144(6):1219-1223

Togliatto M, Carrozzo M, Conrotto D, Pagano M, Gandolfo S Oral lupus erythematosus. Description and analysis of 11 cases. Minerva Stomatol 2000 Jan-Feb; 49(1-2):35-40

Lymphangioma

Clinical features

Colourless, sometimes finely nodular soft mass mainly on the tongue, lips, and buccal mucosa. Bleeding into lymphatic spaces causes sudden purplish discolouration. In the tongue it may cause macroglossia. In the lip, it may cause macrocheilia.

Incidence

Rare.

Aetiology

Hamartoma or benign neoplasm of lymphatic channels.

Diagnosis

Excision biopsy.

Differentiate from haemangiomas mainly.

Management

Excise.

References

Brennan TD, Miller AS, Chen SY Lymphangiomas of the oral cavity: a clinicopathologic, immuno-histochemical, and electron-microscopic study. J Oral Maxillofac Surg 1997 Sep; 55(9):932-935

Sato M, Tanaka N, Sato T, Amagasa T Oral and maxillofacial tumours in children: a review. Br J Oral Maxillofac Surg 1997 Apr; 35(2):92-95

Lymphomas (Non-Hodgkin's)

Clinical features

Oral manifestations may be part of disseminated disease or the only manifestation. In disseminated disease the onset can be fulminant or quiet and the presenting symptoms usually represented by a painless lymphadenopathy (cervical, axillary and inguinal), weight loss and fever.

In the oral cavity, appears as a painless swelling and in the advanced phases it may ulcerate.

Incidence

Uncommon, but mainly seen in HIV/AIDS disease.

Aetiology

Unknown.

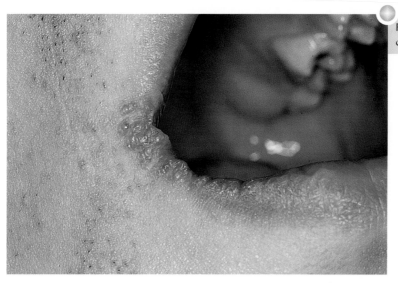

FIGURE 4.120 Lymphangioma. Small commissural soft nodules.

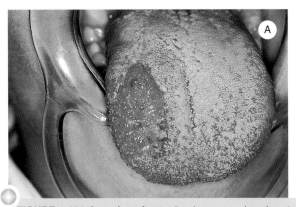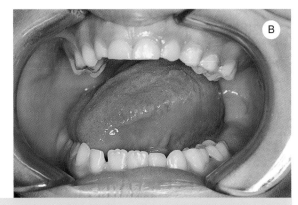

FIGURE 4.121 **Lymphangioma.** On the tongue, lymphangiomas may resemble fungiform papillae (A) or they may cause unilateral macroglossia (B).

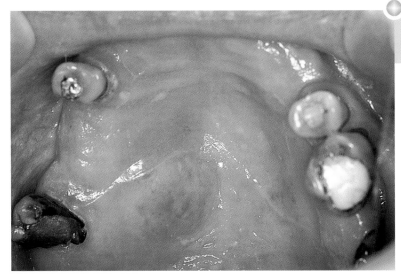

FIGURE 4.122 **Non-Hodgkin lymphoma.** Painless, rapidly growing palatal swelling.

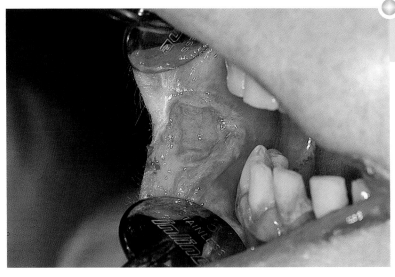

FIGURE 4.123 **Non-Hodgkin lymphoma.** Rarely, oral lymphomas may appear as deep ulcerations.

Diagnosis

Biopsy, histologic examination and immunotyping of the infiltrating cell.

Differentiate from salivary gland tumours, the ulcers must be differentiated from major apthae or squamous cell carcinoma.

Management

Radiotherapy or chemotherapy.

References

Castellano S, Carbone M, Carrozzo M, Broccoletti R, Pagano M, Vasino MA, Gandolfo S Onset of oral extranodal large B-cell non-Hodgkin's lymphoma in a patient with polycythemia vera: a rare presentation. Oral Oncol 2002 Sep; 38(6):624-626

Nocini P, Lo Muzio L, Fior A, Staibano S, Mignogna MD Primary non-Hodgkin's lymphoma of the jaws: immunohistochemical and genetic review of 10 cases. J Oral Maxillofac Surg 2000 Jun; 58(6): 636-644

Richards A, Costelloe MA, Eveson JW, Scully C, Irvine GH, Rooney N Oral mucosal non-Hodgkin's lymphoma - a dangerous mimic. Oral Oncol 2000 Nov 1; 36(6):556-558

Measles

Clinical features

Incubation period is 7-14 days. Koplik's spots - small white spots on the buccal mucosa during prodrome. Maculopapular rash, conjunctivitis, runny nose, cough, fever, malaise and anorexia may be seen.

Incidence

Common childhood exanthem.

Aetiology

Measles virus.

Diagnosis

Clinical features. Rising antibody titre confirmatory.

Differentiate from thrush, Fordyce spots (not in children).

Management

Symptomatic (see herpes simplex).

References

Katz J, Guelmann M, Stavropolous F, Heft M Gingival and other oral manifestations in measles virus infection. J Clin Periodontol 2003 Jul; 30(7):665-668

Scully C, Laskaris G Mucocutaneous disorders. Periodontol 2000. 1998 Oct; 18:81-94

Median Rhomboid Glossitis

Clinical features

Rhomboidal (diamond-shaped) or elliptical reddish, smooth or nodular surface located in the midline of the dorsum of the tongue anterior to the circumvallate papillae.

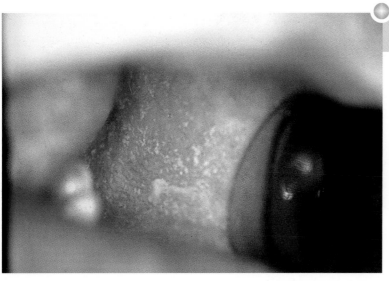

FIGURE 4.124 **Measles.** Koplik's spots.

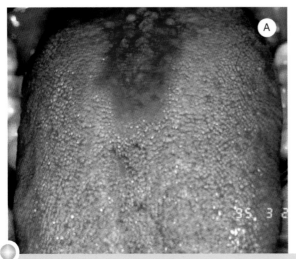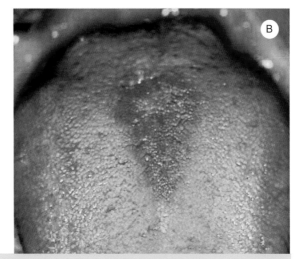

FIGURE 4.125 **Median rhomboid glossitis.** Two typical appearances: median red lesions (A) with a rhomboid outline (B).

Incidence

Uncommon.

Aetiology

Was once thought to be a developmental anomaly (caused by the persistence of tuberculum impar) but it is now thought to be related to localised candidosis.

Diagnosis

Clinical features. Smear and Gram stain for *Candida*.

Management

Antifungals if candidal.

References

McCullough MJ, Savage NW Oral candidosis and the therapeutic use of antifungal agents in dentistry. Aust Dent J 2005 Dec; 50(4 Suppl 2):S36-S39

Zegarelli DJ Fungal infections of the oral cavity. Otolaryngol Clin North Am 1993 Dec; 26(6):1069-1089

Mucocele

Clinical features

Dome-shaped, bluish, translucent, fluctuant painless swelling, usually ≤1 cm in diameter. They rupture easily to release viscid salty mucus, but frequently recur.

Incidence

Common: mostly inside the lower lip and in young adults/children, particularly males. Sometimes seen in buccal mucosa, palate or floor of mouth.

Aetiology

Usually extravasation of mucus from damaged salivary gland duct; rarely retention of mucus within a salivary gland or duct.

Diagnosis

Microscopic features.

Diagnosis is clearcut but a salivary gland neoplasm must be excluded, particularly in cystic swellings in *upper* lip.

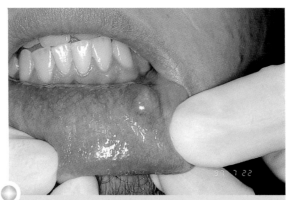

FIGURE 4.126 **Mucocele** of the lip.

Management

If asymptomatic and small, observe; otherwise, use cryosurgery or excision.

References

Esmeili T, Lozada-Nur F, Epstein J Common benign oral soft tissue masses. Dent Clin North Am 2005 Jan; 49(1):223-240

Bodner L, Tal H Salivary gland cysts of the oral cavity: clinical observation and surgical management. Compendium 1991 Mar; 12(3):150, 152, 154-156

Porter SR, Scully C, Kainth B, Ward-Booth P Multiple salivary mucoceles in a young boy. Int J Paediatr Dent 1998 Jun; 8(2):149-151

Mumps
(Acute viral parotitis)

Clinical features

Incubation period is 14-21 days. Malaise, fever, anorexia and sialadenitis - painful, diffuse swelling of one/both parotids and sometimes submandibulars. Saliva is non-purulent; the duct is inflamed. Also trismus and dry mouth.

Complications are uncommon, but include pancreatitis, encephalitis, orchitis, oophoritis and deafness.

Incidence

Fairly common: typically in children.

Aetiology

Mumps virus; rarely Coxsackie, ECHO, EBV or HIV infection.

Diagnosis

Clinical. Mumps antibody titres rarely needed; serum amylase or lipase (occasionally).

Differentiate from obstructive and/or bacterial sialadenitis mainly.

Management

Symptomatic.

References

Bradley PJ Benign salivary gland disease. Hosp Med 2001 Jul; 62(7):392-395

McQuone SJ Acute viral and bacterial infections of the salivary glands. Otolaryngol Clin North Am 1999 Oct; 32(5):793-811

Naevi

Clinical features

Brownish or bluish macules, usually <1 cm across. Asymptomatic.

Incidence

Not known.

Aetiology

Congenital.

Diagnosis

Biopsy.

Differentiate from other causes of pigmentation, especially amalgam tattoo or melanoma.

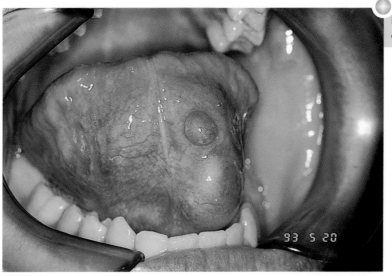

FIGURE 4.127 **Mucocele** of the floor of the mouth.

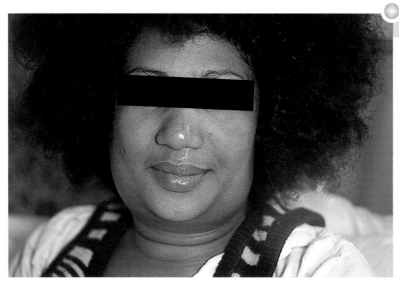

FIGURE 4.128 **Mumps.**

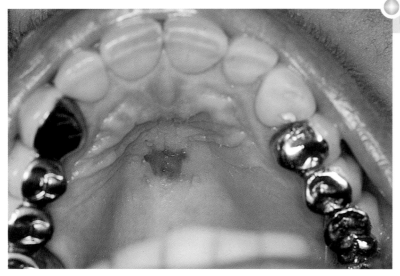

FIGURE 4.129 **Naevus** of the palate.

Management

Excision biopsy to exclude malignant melanoma.

References

Cicek Y, Ertas U The normal and pathological pigmentation of oral mucous membrane: a review. J Contemp Dent Pract 2003 Aug 15; 4(3):76-86

Fistarol SK, Itin PH Plaque-type blue nevus of the oral cavity. Dermatology 2005; 211(3):224-233

Hatch CL Pigmented lesions of the oral cavity. Dent Clin North Am 2005 Jan; 49(1):185-201

Kauzman A, Pavone M, Blanas N, Bradley G Pigmented lesions of the oral cavity: review, differential diagnosis, and case presentations. J Can Dent Assoc 2004 Nov; 70(10):682-683

Necrotising Sialometaplasia

Clinical features

The initial lesion is a nodular swelling usually seen in the posterior part of the hard palate that later leads to a painful craterlike ulcer with irregular border.

Incidence

Rare.

Aetiology

Unknown.

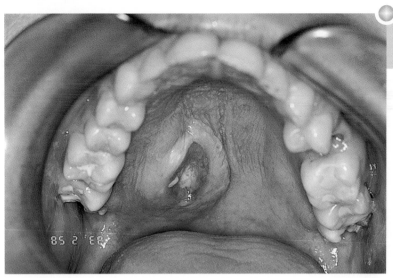

FIGURE 4.130 Necrotising sialometaplasia. Deep, painful ulcer.

Diagnosis

Biopsy is often required to differentiate from malignant salivary gland tumours and squamous cell carcinoma.

Management

Reassurance. The lesions usually heal spontaneously without treatment over 4 to 10 weeks.

References

Imbery TA, Edwards PA Necrotising sialometaplasia: literature review and case reports. J Am Dent Assoc 1996; 127(7):1087-1092

Lombardi T, Samson J, Kuffer R Subacute necrotizing sialadenitis: a form of necrotizing sialometaplasia? Arch Otolaryngol Head Neck Surg 2003 Sep; 129(9):972-975

Scully C, Eveson J Sialosis and necrotising sialometaplasia in bulimia; a case report. Int J Oral Maxillofac Surg 2004 Dec; 33(8):808-810

Necrotising Ulcerative Gingivitis

Clinical features

Acute inflammatory gingival disease characterised by destruction of one or more interdental papillae and rapid destruction of gingiva.

Necrotic lesions start from the gingival margin.

Pain, unpleasant halitosis, bleeding and a pseudomembrane are usually present.

Malaise, fever and cervical lymphadenitis are rare.

Incidence

Uncommon, except in lower socioeconomic groups and in HIV/AIDS.

Aetiology

Fuso-spirochaetal flora, poor oral hygiene, previous marginal gingivitis or periodontitis, smoking and mental or physical stress.

It is more common in HIV seropositives than in general population (see: *Lesions strongly associated with HIV infection*).

Diagnosis

Clinical signs.

Management

In the acute phase: oral hygiene instruction, maintenance of optimal supragingival plaque control mechanically and chemically (chlorhexidine mouth rinses). Metronidazole 200 mg three times a day for 1 week

Professional control is of paramount importance to prevent recurrent disease.

References

Bermejo-Fenoll A, Sanchez-Perez A Necrotising periodontal diseases. Med Oral Patol Oral Cir Bucal 2004; 9 Suppl: 114-119; 108-114

Folayan MO Epidemiology, etiology, and pathophysiology of acute necrotizing ulcerative

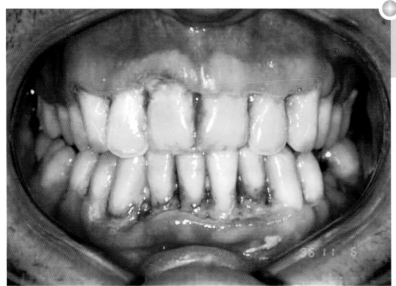

FIGURE 4.131 Necrotising gingivitis. Note the necrosis of interdental papillae of the lower anterior area and the upper gingivae in a HIV-positive patient.

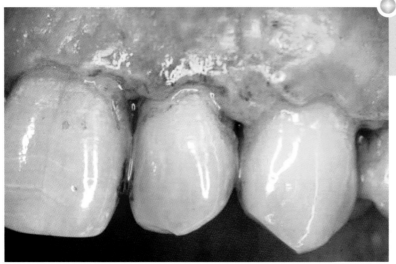

FIGURE 4.132 Necrotising gingivitis. Close view of an HIV-negative patient with other risk factors also (smoking, poor oral hygiene, fatigue and stress).

gingivitis associated with malnutrition. J Contemp Dent Pract 2004 Aug 15; 5(3):28-41

Jones AC, Gulley ML, Freedman PD Necrotising ulcerative stomatitis in human immunodeficiency virus-seropositive individuals: a review of the histopathologic, immunohistochemical, and virologic characteristics of 18 cases. Oral Surg Oral Med Oral Pathol Oral Radiol Endod 2000 Mar; 89(3):323-332

Salama C, Finch D, Bottone EJ Fusospirochetosis causing necrotic oral ulcers in patients with HIV infection. Oral Surg Oral Med Oral Pathol Oral Radiol Endod 2004 Sep; 98(3):321-323

Palatal Papillary Hyperplasia

Clinical features

Typically involves the palate with painless multiple erythematous and oedematous papillary projections tightly aggregated producing an overall verrucous appearance; most frequently involved is the vault, less commonly the alveolar ridge or the palatal incline.

Other oral candidosis (angular stomatitis, denture-related stomatitis) are often present.

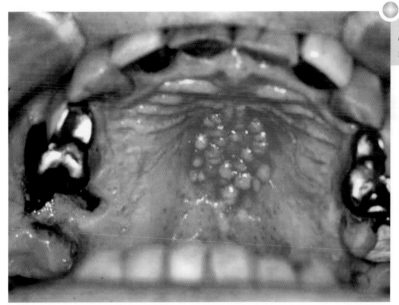

FIGURE 4.133 Papillary hyperplasia of the palate. Uncommon manifestation in a dentate patient.

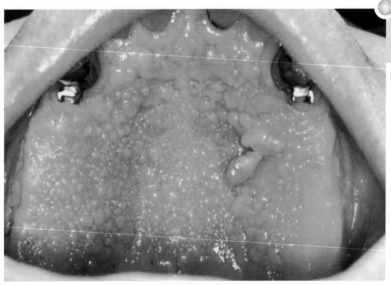

FIGURE 4.134 Papillary hyperplasia of the palate. Involvement of the entire palate in a denture-wearing patient.

Incidence

Common.

Aetiology

Appears to be associated with ill-fitting or loose dentures that predispose to, or potentiate growth of, *Candida albicans*.

Diagnosis

Clinical. Smear for hyphae.

Differentiate from carcinoma or erythroplasia.

Management

In mild cases, leave dentures out at night in antifungal. Antifungal therapy and soft tissue-conditioning agents can produce sufficient resolution to preclude surgery.

Surgical removal is indicated in failed treatment or in severe cases.

References

Antonelli JR, Panno FV, Witko A Inflammatory papillary hyperplasia: supraperiosteal excision by the blade-loop technique. Gen Dent 1998 Jul-Aug; 46(4):390-397

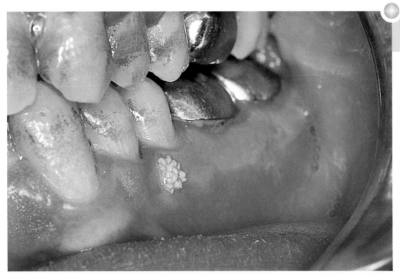

FIGURE 4.135 Papilloma of the gingiva.

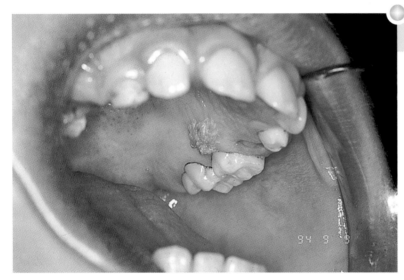

FIGURE 4.136 Papilloma of the hard palate.

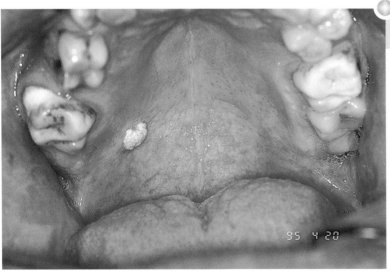

FIGURE 4.137 Papilloma of the soft palate.

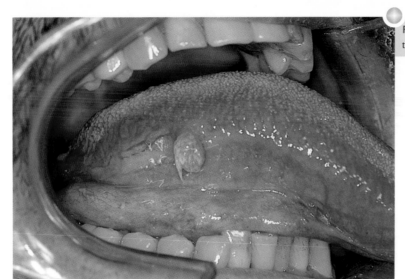

FIGURE 4.138 **Papilloma** of the tongue border.

Kaplan I, Vered M, Moskona D, Buchner A, Dayan D An immunohistochemical study of p53 and PCNA in inflammatory papillary hyperplasia of the palate: a dilemma of interpretation. Oral Dis 1998 Sep; 4(3):194-199

Salonen MA, Raustia AM, Oikarinen KS Effect of treatment of palatal inflammatory papillary hyperplasia with local and systemic antifungal agents accompanied by renewal of complete dentures. Acta Odontol Scand 1996 Apr; 54(2):87-91

Papillomas

Clinical features

Most commonly papillated asymptomatic, pedunculated lesions, either pink or white, on the palate, tongue or other sites (lip, gingiva, buccal mucosa).

Incidence

Most common benign soft tissue neoplasm. Typically in 20-50 year age group.

Aetiology

Human papillomaviruses (HPV).

HPV are also implicated in various warts including venereal warts (condyloma acuminatum), and rare disorders, e.g. focal epithelial hyperplasia (Heck's disease).

Diagnosis

Clinical. Biopsy.

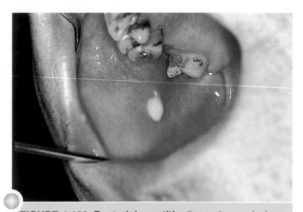

FIGURE 4.139 **Bacterial parotitis.** Pus at Stenson's duct orifice.

Mainly from warts and other epithelial neoplasms.

Management

Excise and microscopic examination; topical podophyllin, imiquimod or intralesional alpha interferon.

References

Fox PA, Tung MY Human papillomavirus: burden of illness and treatment cost considerations. Am J Clin Dermatol 2005; 6(6):399-413

Miller CS, White DK Human papillomavirus expression in oral mucosa, premalignant conditions, and squamous cell carcinoma: a retrospective review of the literature. Oral Surg Oral Med Oral Pathol Oral Radiol Endod 1996 Jul; 82(1):57-68

Praetorius S HPV-associated diseases of oral mucosa. Clin Dermatol 1997 May-Jun; 15(3):399-413

Parotitis

Clinical features

Painful swelling of one gland only, with red, shiny overlying skin, trismus, and purulent discharge from duct.

Incidence

Rare, except in association with xerostomia.

Aetiology

Usually a bacterial infection ascends the duct of a non-functioning gland. Infectious agents include pneumococci, *Staphylococcus aureus* or viridans streptococci.

Diagnosis

Clinical. Pus for culture and sensitivities.

Differentiate mainly from mumps.

Management

Antimicrobials (flucloxacillin if staphylococcus and not allergic to penicillin); analgesics; sialogogues.

References

Scully C An update on recent advances in the understanding of non-neoplastic diseases of the salivary glands. Br J Oral Maxillofac Surg 1992 Aug; 30(4):244-247

Scully C, Porter SR Orofacial disease: update for the dental clinical team: 8. Salivary complaints. Dent Update 1999 Oct; 26(8):357-365

Scully C An update on recent advances in the understanding of non-neoplastic diseases of the salivary glands. Br J Oral Maxillofac Surg 1992 Aug; 30(4):244-247

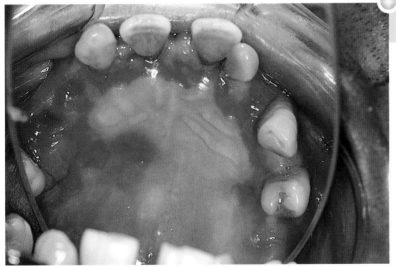

FIGURE 4.140 **Mucous membrane pemphigoid**. Desquamative gingivitis

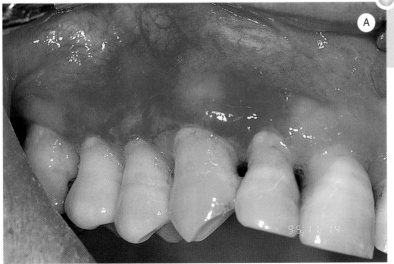

FIGURE 4.141 **Mucous membrane pemphigoid**. Erosive gingival pemphigoid (A). It is sometimes also possible to observe intact blisters (B, C).

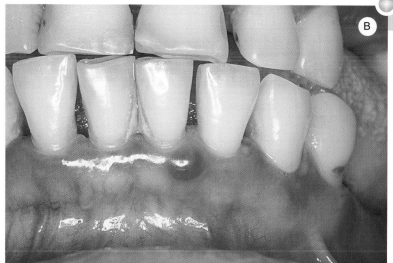

FIGURE 4.141 *Continued.*

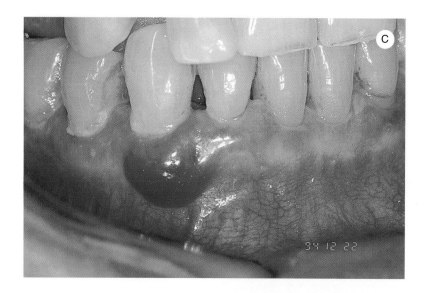

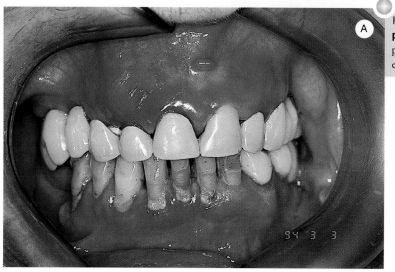

FIGURE 4.142 **Mucous membrane pemphigoid.** Gingival features of pemphigoid with erythematous (A) and erosive areas (B, C).

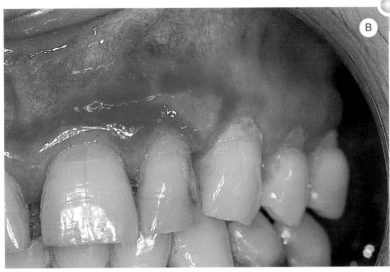

FIGURE 4.142 *Continued.*

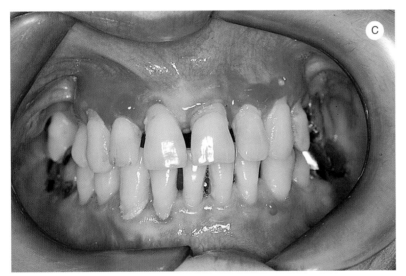

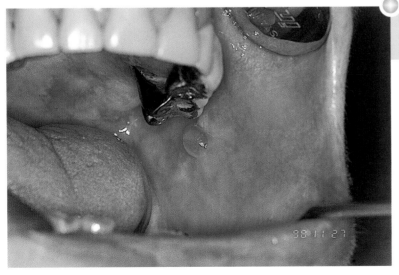

FIGURE 4.143 Mucous membrane pemphigoid. Intact blister of the left buccal mucosa.

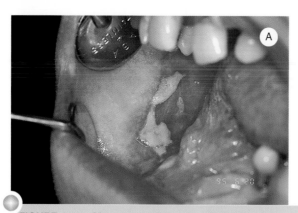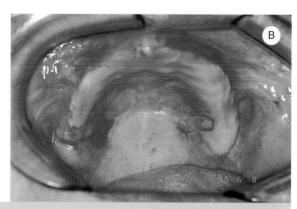

FIGURE 4.144 Mucous membrane pemphigoid. Fibrin-covered yellow erosions (A, B) are the most characteristic lesions of oral pemphigoid after desquamative gingivitis.

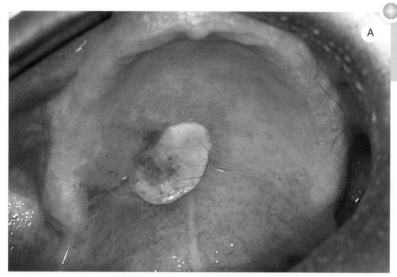

FIGURE 4.145 Mucous membrane pemphigoid. Broken blister of the palate (A) and severe ulceration of the pharynx (B).

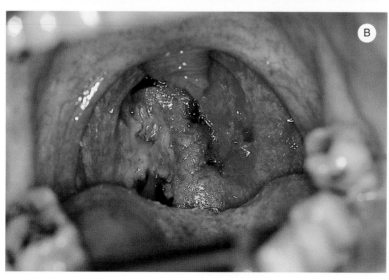

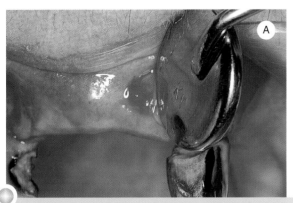
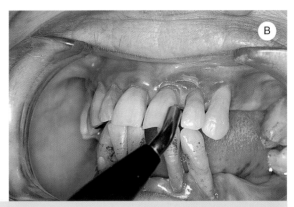

FIGURE 4.146 Mucous membrane pemphigoid. Nikolsky's sign: gentle massage of clinically uninvolved sites may produce a blister or desquamation (A). This may be created by an air blast (B).

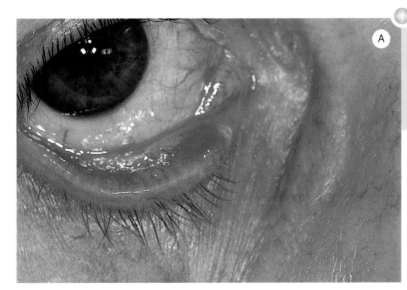

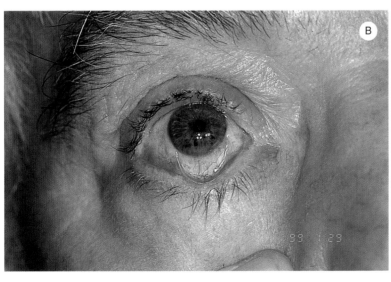

FIGURE 4.147 Mucous membrane pemphigoid. Ocular lesions: at the beginning, an erythematous-erosive conjunctivitis may be seen (A). Scarring following repeated fibrosis can lead to the fusion of the scleral and palpebral conjunctivae (symblepharon) (B).

Pemphigoid, Mucous Membrane

Clinical features

Oral: blisters (sometimes blood-filled) can present anywhere, but especially at sites of trauma. Nikolsky's sign may be positive. Ulcers follow blisters and may heal with scarring. 'Desquamative gingivitis' is common.

Others: *conjunctival lesions* - leading to impaired sight (entropion or symblepharon)

laryngeal lesions - may lead to stenosis

skin lesions - blisters rarely.
genital lesions

Incidence

Not uncommon: mainly in middle-aged or elderly females.

Aetiology

Autoimmune.

Diagnosis

Biopsy - subepithelial split, including immuno-fluorescence (C_3 and IgG at basement membrane).

Differentiate from other causes of mouth ulcers, especially pemphigus and localised oral purpura. The 'desquamative gingivitis' must be differentiated from lichen planus.

Management

Potent topical corticosteroids, tacrolimus or, rarely, systemic corticosteroids or dapsone.

References

Carbone M, Carrozzo M, Castellano S, Conrotto D, Broccoletti R, Gandolfo S Systemic corticosteroid therapy of oral vesiculoerosive diseases (OVED). An open trial. Minerva Stomatol 1998; 47(10):479-487

Carrozzo M, Cozzani E, Broccoletti R, Carbone M, Pentenero M, Arduino P, Parodi A, Gandolfo S Analysis of antigens targeted by circulating IgG and IgA antibodies in patients with mucous membrane pemphigoid predominantly affecting the oral cavity. J Periodontol 2004 Oct; 75(10):1302-1308

Carrozzo M, Fasano ME, Broccoletti R, Carbone M, Cozzani E, Rendine S, Roggero S, Parodi A,

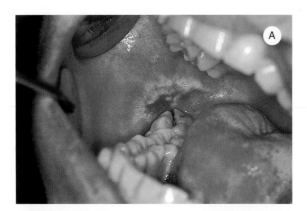

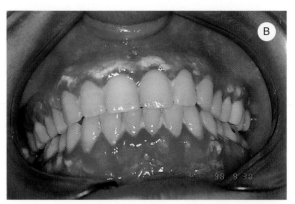

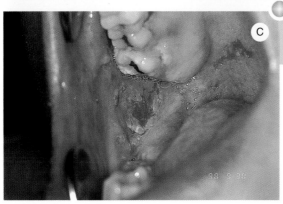

FIGURE 4.148 Pemphigus vulgaris. The first manifestation of pemphigus may often be red oral erosions (A, C) or desquamative gingivitis (B).

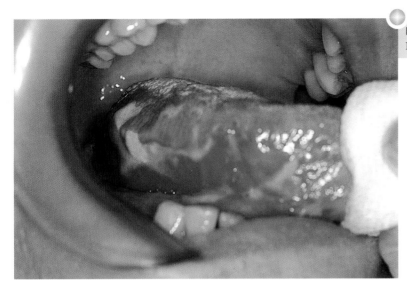

FIGURE 4.149 Pemphigus vulgaris.
Lingual lesions of pemphigus.

Gandolfo S HLA-DQB1 alleles in Italian patients with mucous membrane pemphigoid predominantly affecting the oral cavity. Br J Dermatol 2001 Nov; 145(5):805-808

Scully C, Carrozzo M, Gandolfo S, Puiatti P, Monteil R Update on mucous membrane pemphigoid: a heterogeneous immune-mediated subepithelial blistering entity. Oral Surg Oral Med Oral Pathol Oral Radiol Endod 1999; 88(1):56-68

Pemphigus Vulgaris

Clinical features

Oral lesions often precede skin lesions. Blisters anywhere on the mucosa (most frequently palate, gingiva and buccal mucosa) rupture rapidly to leave ragged ulcers. Nikolsky's sign is positive.

Skin lesions: large flaccid blisters especially where there is trauma.

Other lesions: conjunctivae or genitals particularly.

Pemphigus is lethal if not treated.

Incidence

Rare. It is mainly a disease of middle-aged women, especially from around the Mediterranean and Ashkenazi Jews. HLA-DRG/DRG Association.

Aetiology

Autoimmune: circulating autoantibodies to epithelial intercellular substance.

Diagnosis

Biopsy to show acantholysis, including immunofluorescence to show IgG and C_3 binding to intercellular attachments of epithelial cells.

Serology (antibodies to epithelial intercellular substance (desmoglein)).

Differentiate from other causes of mouth ulcers, especially mucous membrane pemphigoid.

Management

Immunosuppression with systemic corticosteroids plus azathioprine, other immunosuppressives, or gold.

References

Black M, Mignogna MD, Scully C Number II. Pemphigus vulgaris. Oral Dis 2005 May; 11(3): 119-130

Mignogna MD, Lo Muzio L, Mignogna RE, Carbone R, Ruoppo E, Bucci E Oral pemphigus: long term behaviour and clinical response to treatment with deflazacort in sixteen cases. J Oral Pathol Med 2000 Apr; 29(4):145-152

Scully C, Challacombe SJ Pemphigus vulgaris: update on etiopathogenesis, oral manifestations, and management. Crit Rev Oral Biol Med 2002; 13(5):397-408

Scully C, Paes De Almeida O, Porter SR, Gilkes JJ Pemphigus vulgaris: the manifestations and long-term management of 55 patients with oral lesions. Br J Dermatol 1999 Jan; 140(1):84-89

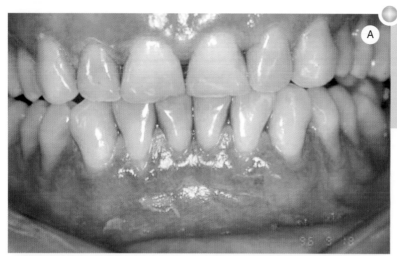

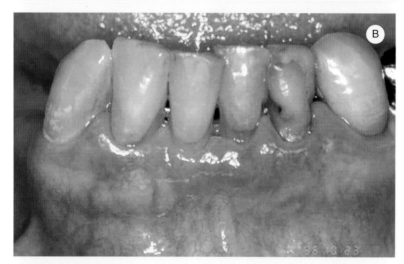

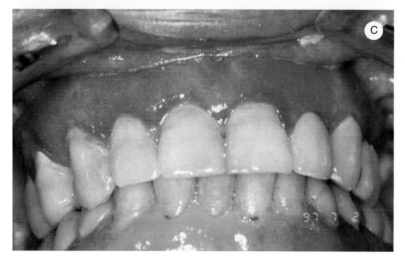

FIGURE 4.150 Plasma cell gingivitis. The clinical appearance resembles that of desquamative gingivitis but the onset is acute, there are no erosions, the colour is more yellow-red (A, B) and it mainly involves the anterior vestibular gingivae (C).

Plasma Cell Gingivitis

Incidence
Uncommon.

Aetiology
Contact allergy: drugs, tooth paste, mouth rinses, topical fluorides, chewing-gum and a numbers of dental materials may produce an allergic response.

Clinical features
Intensely inflammatory hyperemic gingivostomatitis, which may occur in conjunction with angular cheilitis and glossitis

Diagnosis
History and clinical features. Patch-tests.

Differentiate from desquamative gingivitis.

Management
If possible, remove aetiological factors.

References
Hedin CA, Karpe B, Larsson A Plasma-cell gingivitis in children and adults. A clinical and histological description. Swed Dent J 1994; 18(4):117-124

Roman CC, Yuste CM, Gonzalez MA, Gonzalez AP, Lopez G Plasma cell gingivitis. Cutis 2002 Jan; 69(1):41-45

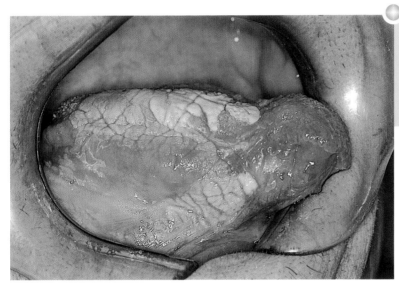

FIGURE 4.151 **Proliferative verrucous leukoplakia.** A 75-year-old woman with multiple white verrucous plaques involving the dorsum and the ventrum of the tongue and both the buccal mucosae (not shown in the figure).

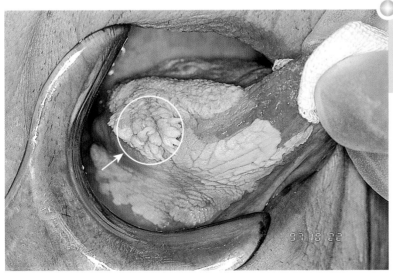

FIGURE 4.152 **Proliferative verrucous leukoplakia.** After 1 year the same patient as Figure 4.151 developed a verrucous carcinoma (arrow).

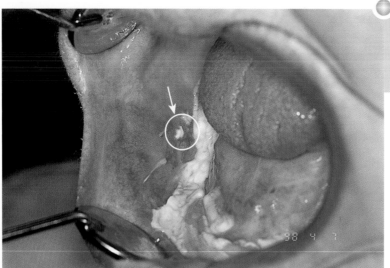

FIGURE 4.153 **Proliferative verrucous leukoplakia.** A 68-year-old woman with long lasting (10 years) oral manifestations: recent onset of an early squamous cell carcinoma (arrow).

Proliferative Verrucous Leukoplakia

Clinical features

Progressively expanding exophytic/verrucal, predominantly white, lesions present in multiple intraoral sites. Lesions begin as a simple hyperkeratosis that spreads locally or to other sites to become multifocal and proliferative.

Associated with a high risk of malignant transformation.

Incidence

Rare: women are affected more frequently than men.

Aetiology

Unknown.

Diagnosis

Early biopsy is mandatory for these lesions.

Management

Surgical excision or laser ablation, but control of PVL is unsatisfactory.

References

Bagan JV, Jimenez Y, Sanchis JM, Poveda R, Milian MA, Murillo J, Scully C Proliferative verrucous leukoplakia: high incidence of gingival squamous cell carcinoma. J Oral Pathol Med 2003 Aug; 32(7): 379-382

Bagan JV, Murillo J, Poveda R, Gavalda C, Jimenez Y, Scully C Proliferative verrucous leukoplakia: unusual locations of oral squamous cell carcinomas, and field cancerization as shown by the appearance of multiple OSCCs. Oral Oncol 2004 Apr; 40(4):440-443

Batsakis JG, Suarez P, el-Naggar AK Proliferative verrucous leukoplakia and its related lesions. Oral Oncol 1999; 35(4):354-359

Campisi G, Giovannelli L, Ammatuna P, Capra G, Colella G, Di Liberto C, Gandolfo S, Pentenero M, Carrozzo M, Serpico R, D'Angelo M Proliferative verrucous vs conventional leukoplakia: no significantly increased risk of HPV infection. Oral Oncol 2004 Sep; 40(8):835-840

Purpura

Clinical features

Red or brown pinpoint lesions (petechiae) or diffuse bruising (ecchymoses) mainly at sites of trauma. Lesions do not blanch on pressure (*c.f.*, haemangioma). Palatal petechiae are a feature of thrombocytopenia, infections, such as infectious mononucleosis, but may be seen in HIV disease or rubella, or where there is trauma such as coughing, or vomiting in bulimia or in fellatio.

Incidence

Occasional small traumatic petechiae at the occlusal line are seen in otherwise healthy patients. Otherwise, oral purpura is uncommon.

Aetiology

Platelet deficiency - idiopathic (autoimmune), sometimes in HIV/AIDS:

- platelet defect
- vascular defect

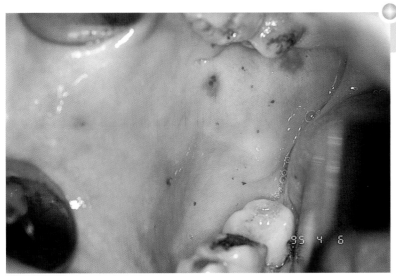

FIGURE 4.154 Purpura. Oral petechiae in a thrombocytopenic patient.

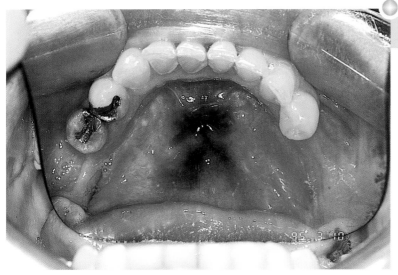

FIGURE 4.155 Purpura. Ecchymoses caused by surgical trauma.

- localised oral purpura ('angina bullosa haemorrhagica').

Diagnosis

Blood picture (including platelet count) and haemostatic function.

Differentiate from haemangiomas, telangiectasia and Kaposi's sarcoma. Thrombocytopenia is also seen in HIV infection.

Management

Treat the underlying cause.

References

Fenner M, Frankenberger R, Pressmar K, John S, Neukam FW, Nkenke E Life-threatening thrombotic thrombocytopenic purpura associated with dental foci. Report of two cases. J Clin Periodontal 2004 Nov; 31(11):1019-1023

Scully C, Felix DH Oral medicine: update for the dental practitioner: red and pigmented lesions. Br Dent J 2005 Nov 26; 199(10):639-645

Themistocleous E, Ariyaratnam S, Duxbury AJ Acute idiopathic thrombocytopenic purpura: a case report. Dent Update 2004 Mar; 31(2):92-96

Localised Oral Purpura
(see Angina bullosa haemorrhagica)

Racial Pigmentation

Clinical features

Brown (rarely black) pigmentation, especially of the gingiva.

Aetiology

Racial pigmentation is seen not only in coloured patients, but also in some whites, especially those from the Mediterranean region.

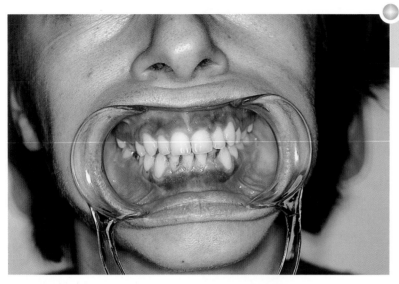

FIGURE 4.156 Racial pigmentation. Diffuse gingival pigmentation in a young Mediterranean woman.

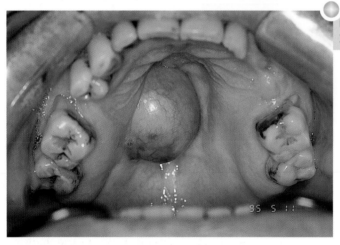

FIGURE 4.157 Salivary gland neoplasms. Pleomorphic adenoma.

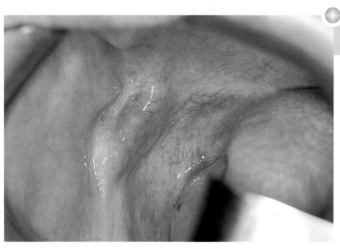

FIGURE 4.158 Salivary gland neoplasms. Adenoid cystic carcinoma.

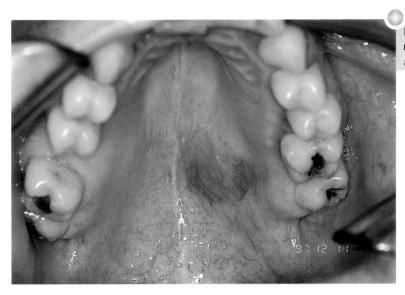

FIGURE 4.159 Salivary gland neoplasms. Low-grade polymorphic adenocarcinoma of the palate.

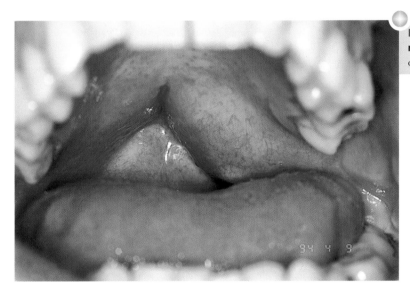

FIGURE 4.160 Salivary gland neoplasms. Adenoid cystic carcinoma of the submandibular gland.

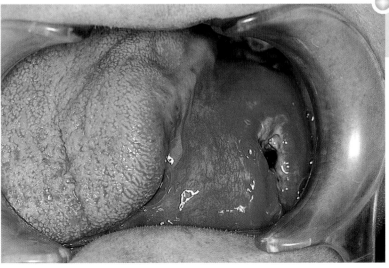

FIGURE 4.161 Salivary gland neoplasms. Myoepithelioma of the palate.

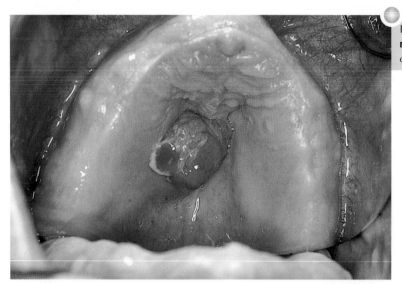

FIGURE 4.162 Salivary gland neoplasms. Terminal duct carcinoma of the palate.

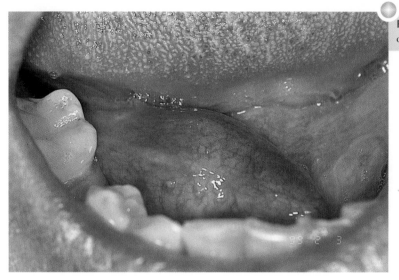

FIGURE 4.163 Salivary obstruction of the Wharton duct caused by calculus.

Incidence

Common: the main cause of oral pigmentation.

Diagnosis

Differentiate from other causes of pigmentation.

Management

Reassure.

References

Scully C, Porter S ABC of oral health. Swellings and red, white, and pigmented lesions. BMJ 2000 Jul 22: 321(7255):225-228

Scully C, Porter SR Orofacial disease: update for the dental clinical team: 4. Red, brown, black and bluish lesions. Dent Update 1999 May; 26(4):169-173

Salivary Neoplasms

Clinical features

Usually pleomorphic adenomas presenting as rubbery and lobulated asymptomatic swelling in one gland (usually parotid). Malignant tumours in late stages are often painful and ulcerate and metastasise to upper cervical lymph nodes. Malignant neoplasms classically grow rapidly, and may involve nerves (e.g. facial palsy).

Classification of salivary neoplasms:
- Adenomas
  pleomorphic
  'monomorphic': adenolymphoma/oncocytic
     adenoma
  others

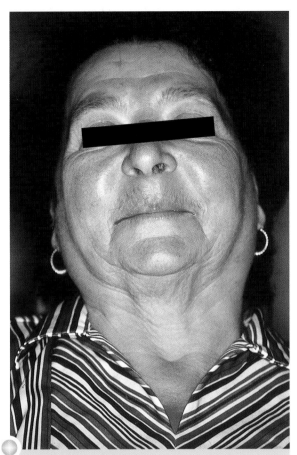

FIGURE 4.164 Sialadenosis.

- Mucoepidermoid carcinoma
- Acinic cell carcinoma
- Adenoid cystic and other carcinomas.

Most common are pleomorphic salivary adenomas, muco-epidermoid tumours and adenoid cystic carcinomas. 75% involve parotid; 60% are pleomorphic salivary adenomas and benign.

Pleomorphic adenoma is the most common *intraoral* salivary neoplasm, but adenoid cystic carcinoma and mucoepidermoid carcinoma are relatively more common in the mouth than in the major glands. The palate is the site of predilection. Tumours in the tongue are usually malignant - especially adenoid cystic carcinoma. Those in the lips are typically benign (pleomorphic or other adenoma). Most sublingual gland tumours are malignant.

Incidence

Rare: mainly in middle and old age.

Aetiology

Unknown: polyoma viruses have been implicated in animal models, other viruses, such as EBV, and irradiation in some human neoplasms.

Diagnosis

Microscopy after gland excision (biopsy allows seeding and recurrence).

Differentiate from non-neoplastic salivary gland swellings.

Management

Surgical excision; radiotherapy also for some.

References

Califano J, Eisele DW Benign salivary gland neoplasms. Otolaryngol Clin North Am 1999 Oct; 32(5):861-873

Day TA, Deveikis J, Gillespie MB, Joe JK, Ogretmen B, Osguthorpe JD, Reed SG, Richardson MS, Rossi M, Saini R, Sharma AK, Stuart RK Salivary gland neoplasms. Curr Treat Options Oncol 2004 Feb; 5(1):11-26

Gold DR, Annino DJ Jr Management of the neck in salivary gland carcinoma. Otolaryngol Clin North Am 2005 Feb; 38(1):99-105

Rice DH Malignant salivary gland neoplasms. Otolaryngol Clin North Am 1999 Oct; 32(5):875-886

Salivary Obstruction

Clinical features

Typically there is pain and swelling of a salivary gland at meal times. May be asymptomatic. Obstruction of minor salivary gland duct may produce a mucocele.

Incidence

Fairly common in submandibular duct or gland.

Aetiology

Calculus usually; rarely mucus plug, fibrous stricture or neoplasm.

Diagnosis

Radiography (but 40% of stones are radiolucent); sialography if necessary.

Differentiate from other causes of salivary swelling.

Management

Surgical or lithotripsy removal.

References

Hebert G, Ouimet-Oliva D, Nicolet V, Bourdon F
Imaging of the salivary glands. Can Assoc Radiol J
1993 Oct; 44(5):342-349

Raymond AK, Batsakis JG Angiolithiasis and
sialolithiasis in the head and neck. Ann Otol Rhinol
Laryngol 1992 May: 101(5):455-457

Rice DH Noninflammatory, non-neoplastic disorders
of the salivary glands. Otolaryngol Clin North Am
1999 Oct; 32(5):835-843

Sialosis

Clinical features

Painless bilateral swelling, typically of parotids.

Incidence

Uncommon.

Aetiology

The common feature is autonomic neuropathy.
Known causes include:

- *Neurogenic*: various drugs such as
  isoprenaline
- *Dystrophic-metabolic*: anorexia-bulimia,
  alcoholic cirrhosis, diabetes, malnutrition,
  thyroid disease, acromegaly and pregnancy.

The condition is frequently idiopathic.

Diagnosis

Clinical. Blood glucose, liver function tests,
possibly growth hormone levels.

Management

Exclude and treat predisposing causes.

References

Mignogna MD, Fedele S, Lo Russo L
Anorexia/bulimia-related sialadenosis of palatal minor
salivary glands. J Oral Pathol Med 2004 Aug;
33(7):441-442

Pape SA, MacLeod RI, McLean NR, Soames JV
Sialadenosis of the salivary glands. Br J Plast Surg
1995 Sep; 48(6):419-422

Sjögren's Syndrome

Clinical features

Dry eyes (keratoconjunctivitis sicca): initially
asymptomatic, later gritty sensation, itching,
soreness or inability to cry. Salivary and lacrimal
glands may swell. Dry mouth (xerostomia):
difficulty in eating dry foods, disturbed taste,
speech and swallowing, rampant caries, candidosis
and acute sialadenitis. Saliva is frothy and not
pooling; parchment-like mucosa and lobulated
depapillated tongue. There is no connective tissue
disease in primary Sjögren's syndrome, but it is
present in secondary: typically rheumatoid
arthritis or primary biliary cirrhosis, and
occasionally other autoimmune disorders. A
similar syndrome may be seen in HIV disease.

Incidence

Uncommon: mainly middle-aged or elderly women.

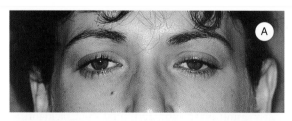
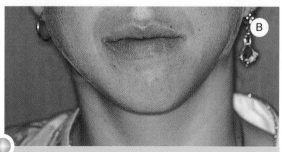

FIGURE 4.165 Sjögren's syndrome. In a young
woman; note the dry eyes and mouth.

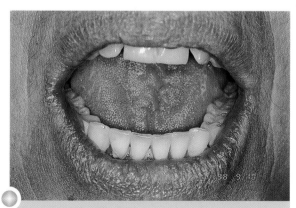

FIGURE 4.166 Sjögren's syndrome. Dry mouth.

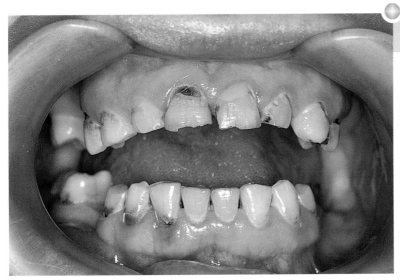

FIGURE 4.167 Sjögren's syndrome.
Diffuse dental caries.

Aetiology

Autoimmune inflammatory exocrinopathy. There may be a viral aetiology and a genetic predisposition.

Diagnosis

Clinical. Ro (SS-A), La (SS-B) and other autoantibodies, especially rheumatoid factor. Salivary flow rates reduced. Labial gland biopsy, sialography and/or scintigraphy or ultrasonography.

Differentiate from other causes of xerostomia, especially drugs (anticholinergics such as tricyclic antidepressants and sympathomimetics), dehydration, HIV salivary gland disease, irradiation, sarcoidosis.

Management

Control underlying disease: at present experimental (e.g. ciclosporin).

Eyes - methylcellulose eye drops or rarely ligation or cautery of nasolacrimal duct.

Dry mouth - preventive dental care (oral hygiene, limitation of sucrose intake, fluorides, chlorhexidine, xylitol-containing chewing gum)

Treat infections.

Sialogogues and/or salivary substitutes (e.g. methylcellulose). Pilocarpine, cevimeline or bethanechol may be used to stimulate salivation.

References

Fox RI Sjogren's syndrome. Lancet 2005 Jul 23-29; 366(9482):321-331

Fox RI Sjogren's syndrome: current therapies remain inadequate for a common disease. Expert Opin Investig Drugs 2000 Sep; 9(9):2007-2016

Hansen A, Lipsky PE, Dorner T Immunopathogenesis of primary Sjogren's syndrome: implications for disease management and therapy. Curr Opin Rheumatol 2005 Sep; 17(5):558-565

Porter SR, Scully C, Hegarty AM An update of the etiology and management of xerostomia. Oral Surg Oral Med Oral Pathol Oral Radiol Endod 2004 Jan; 97(1):28-46

Ramos-Casals M, Font J Primary Sjogren's syndrome: current and emergent aetiopathogenic concepts. Rheumatology (Oxford). 2005 Nov; 44(11):1354-1367

Scully C, Porter SR Orofacial disease: update for the dental clinical team: 8. Salivary complaints. Dent Update 1999; 26(8):357-365

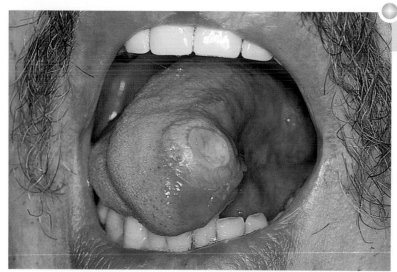

FIGURE 4.168 Syphilis. Primary syphilis of the tongue.

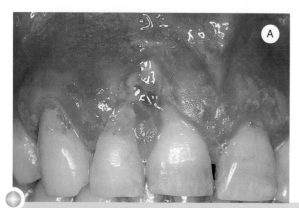 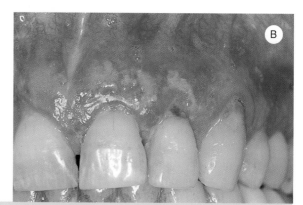

FIGURE 4.169 Syphilis. Gingival mucosal patches of secondary syphilis (A, B).

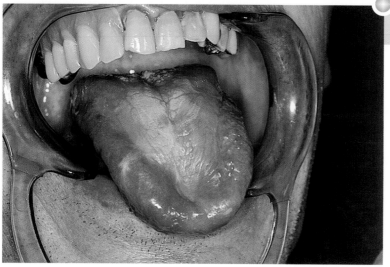

FIGURE 4.170 Syphilis. Lingual lesions.

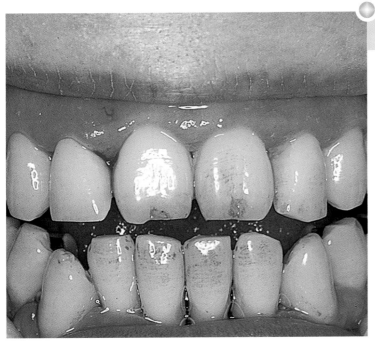

FIGURE 4.171 **Syphilis.** Hutchinson's teeth.

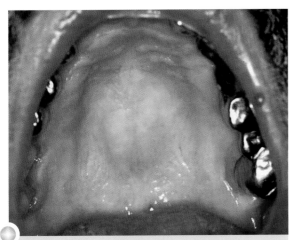

FIGURE 4.172 **Torus palatinus.**

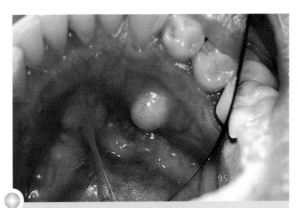

FIGURE 4.173 **Torus mandibularis.**

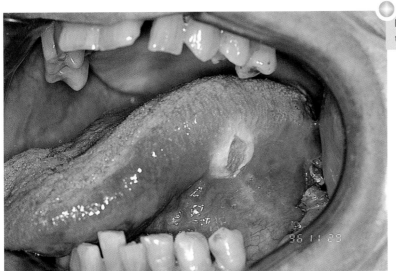

FIGURE 4.174 **Traumatic ulcer.** Note the surrounding white border.

Syphilis

Congenital syphilis

Head and neck: frontal bossing, saddle nose, Hutchinsonian incisors, Moon's or mulberry molars and rhagades.

Others: learning disability, interstitial keratitis, deafness, sabre tibiae and Clutton's joints.

Primary syphilis (Hunterian or hard chancre)

Incubation period is 9-90 days. Small papule develops into large painless indurated ulcer, with regional lymphadenitis. Chancre heals spontaneously in 1-2 months.

Secondary syphilis

Oral lesions are highly infectious: mucous patches, split papules or snail-track ulcers. Rash (coppery coloured typically on palms and soles), condylomata lata and generalised lymph node enlargement.

Tertiary syphilis

Oral lesions are non-infectious: glossitis (leukoplakia) and gumma (usually midline in palate or tongue.

May be cardiovascular complications (aortic aneurysm) or neurosyphilis (tabes dorsalis, general paralysis of the insane, Argyll-Robinson pupils).

Incidence

Uncommon. Predominantly an infection of the sexually promiscuous (prostitutes, male homosexuals, travellers, armed forces).

Aetiology

Treponema pallidum. Sexually transmitted. Other treponematoses, including yaws, bejel and pinta, are rare in the UK.

Diagnosis

T. pallidum in direct smear of primary and secondary stage lesions (darkfield examination). Serology is positive late in primary stage.

Differentiate from trauma, herpes labialis, pyogenic granuloma, carcinoma. Very rarely: non-venereal treponematoses.

Management

Penicillin (depot injection); if allergic to penicillin, use erythromycin or tetracycline.

References

Alam F, Argiriadou AS, Hodgson TA, Kumar N, Porter SR Primary syphilis remains a cause of oral ulceration. Br Dent J 2000 Oct 14: 189(7):352-354

Aquilina C, Viraben R, Denis P Secondary syphilis simulating oral hairy leukoplakia. J Am Acad Dermatol 2003 Oct; 49(4):749-751

Scott CM, Flint SR Oral syphilis: re-emergence of an old disease with oral manifestations. Int J Oral Maxillofac Surg 2005 Jan; 34(1):58-63

Torus Palatinus and Mandibularis

Clinical features

Torus palatinus: a bony exostosis in the midline of hard palate. The size is variable, as is the shape that may be lobular, nodular or irregular. *Torus*

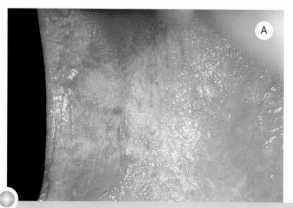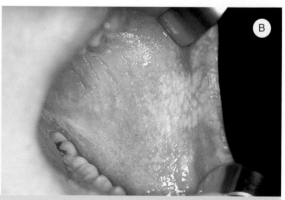

FIGURE 4.175 White sponge naevus. The whole buccal mucosae have a white appearance with a spongy consistency.

mandibularis are bony lumps usually lingual to premolars mainly bilateral located.

Incidence

The incidence is about 20 % and 6% for the palatinus and the mandibular, respectively. Torus is common in the Mongoloid race.

Aetiology

Genetic.

Diagnosis

Clinical (sometime radiography).

Management

No treatment is needed but they may be surgically excised or reduced if a total or partial denture is requested.

References

Chohayeb AA, Volpe AR Occurrence of torus palatinus and mandibularis among women of different ethnic groups. Am J Dent 2001 Oct; 14(5):278-280

Jainkittivong A, Langlais RP Buccal and palatal exostoses: prevalence and concurrence with tori. Oral Surg Oral Med Oral Pathol Oral Radiol Endod 2000 Jul; 90(1):48-53

Traumatic Ulcers

Clinical features

Usually a single ulcer closely related to cause.

Chronic irritation may cause hyperplasia and hyperkeratosis.

Incidence

Common.

Aetiology

Broken teeth, carious teeth, dental prostheses, orthodontic appliances (consider the possibility of a self-inflicted injury).

Diagnosis

Clinical evidence of trauma and healing in few days.

Differentiate from mouth ulcer particularly malignant lesions.

Management

Remove aetiological factors. Local treatment: chlorhexidine mouthwash.

References

Campisi G, Margiotta V Oral mucosal lesions and risk habits among men in an Italian study population. J Oral Pathol Med 2001; 30(1):22-28

Kvam E, Bondevik O, Gjerdet NR Traumatic ulcers and pain in adults during orthodontic treatment. Community Dent Oral Epidemiol 1989 Jun; 17(3):154-157

White Sponge Naevus

Clinical features

Asymptomatic, diffuse, bilateral white lesions with shaggy or spongy, wrinkled surface. Usually involves the buccal mucosa, but sometimes the tongue, the floor of the mouth or elsewhere and may involve the pharynx, oesophagus, nose, genitalia and anus.

Incidence

Rare.

Aetiology

Genetic (mutation of keratin 13 and 14) with an autosomal dominant trait. It appears at birth or during childhood but is often recognised only later.

Diagnosis

Clinical. Biopsy is confirmatory.

Management

There is no specific treatment for this condition as it is asymptomatic and benign.

References

Richard G, De Laurenzi V, Didona B, Bale SJ, Compton JG Keratin 13 point mutation underlies the hereditary mucosal epithelial disorder white sponge nevus. Nat Genet 1995 Dec; 11(4):453-455

Rugg EL, McLean WH, Allison WE, et al A mutation in the mucosal keratin K4 is associated with oral white sponge nevus. Nat Genet 1995 Dec; 11(4):450-452

Terrinoni A, Rugg EL, Lane EB, Melino G, Felix DH, Munro CS, McLean WH A novel mutation in the keratin 13 gene causing oral white sponge nevus. J Dent Res 2001 Mar; 80(3):919-923

PartThree

Therapy

Chapter Five

Guide to the main drugs used in the treatment of oral mucosal diseases

Analgesics

Acetylsalicylic acid

Class: Non-steroidal antiinflammatory drug (NSAIDs).

Indications: Mild pain.

Main side effects: Gastric irritation and interference with haemostasis.

Contraindications: Peptic ulcer, bleeding, asthma, paediatric age group, advanced pregnancy, renal diseases, allergy to acetylsalicylic acid.

Interactions: Corticosteroids and other NSAIDs (risk of peptic ulcer), allopurinol (reduces the effects), and oral antidiabetic drugs (increases the effects).

Adult dose: 300-600 mg up to 6 times daily/daily after meals.

Codeine

Class: Opiate.

Indications: Moderate pain.

Main side effects: Nausea, headaches, drowsiness, constipation, and xerostomia.

Contraindications: Hepatic diseases and advanced pregnancy.

Interactions: Antihistamines, antidepressants, hypnotics and sedatives (increase sedative effects), monoamine oxidase inhibitors, alcohol, cocaine and cannabis (serious toxicity), warfarin (bleeding), analgesics (increases the effects), zidovudine (increases toxicity).

Adult dose: 10-60 mg.

Diclofenac

Class: NSAID.

Indications: Moderate pain.

Main side effects: Gastric irritation, nausea.

Contraindications: Peptic ulcer, pregnancy, hypersensitivity to acetylsalicylic acid.

Interactions: Corticosteroids and other NSAIDs (risk of peptic ulcer), lithium (increases plasma levels), ciclosporin (increases renal toxicity).

Adult dose: 25-75 mg, up to twice daily.

Antibacterial Agents

Amoxicillin

Class: Penicillin.

Indications: Oral bacterial infections. *Staphylococcus aureus* is often resistant.

Main side effects: Rare. Diarrhoea, reactions due to hypersensitivity.

Contraindications: Hypersensitivity to penicillin, toxic dermatitis during mononucleosis, cytomegalovirus infection, lymphoid leukaemia, therapy with allopurinol.

Interactions: Probenecid (prolongs blood levels of amoxicillin), hypersensitivity induced by cephalosporin.

Adult dose: 250-500 mg, 8-hourly.

Ampicillin

Class: Penicillin.

Indications: Oral bacterial infections.

Main side effects: Rare. Pain and inflammation of injected area. Nausea, vomiting, diarrhoea, hypersensitivity.

Contraindications: Hypersensitivity.

Interactions: Probenecid (prolongs and extends the blood l levels of ampicillin), allopurinol (skin reactions to the ampicillin).

Adult dose: 250-500 mg, 8-hourly.

Azithromycin

Class: Macrolide.

Indications: Oral bacterial infections.

Main side effects: Rare. Diarrhoea, abdominal pain, nausea, vomiting.

Contraindications: Hypersensitivity to azithromycin and other macrolides, serious hepatic failure.

Interactions: Do not administer with antacids.

Adult dose: 500 mg daily.

Cefadroxil

Class: Cephalosporin. Acts orally.

Indications: Oral bacterial infections.

Main side effects: Rare. Hypersensitivity.

Contraindications: Hypersensitivity.

Adult dose: 1-2 g, 2 times/daily.

Cefazolin

Class: Cephalosporin.

Indications: Oral bacterial infections.

Main side effects: Rare. Localised pain after injection. Hypersensitivity.

Contraindications: Hypersensitivity. Reduce dosage in case of renal failure.

Interactions: Probenecid (prolongs and extends the blood levels of amoxicillin), aminoglycosides and diuretics (increase renal toxicity).

Adult dose: 1-2 g/daily intramuscular or intravenous, 4 times /daily.

Clarithromycin

Class: Macrolide.

Indications: Oral bacterial infections.

Main side effects: Rare. Diarrhoea, abdominal pain, nausea, headaches, skin rash.

Contraindications: Hypersensitivity, pregnancy, during breast-feeding and serious hepatic failure.

Interactions: It increases the blood haematological levels of carbamazepine and theophylline.

Adult dose: 250 mg, 2 times /daily.

Clindamycin

Indications: Serious oral bacterial infections in case of allergy to penicillin.

Main side effects: Nausea, vomiting, diarrhoea, pseudomembranous colitis.

Contraindications: Hypersensitivity.

Interactions: It can enhance the blocking effect of neuromuscular drugs like pancuronium; adverse reaction with erythromycin.

Adult dose: 10-30 mg/kg/daily, 4 times/daily.

Metronidazole

Indications: Acute necrotising gingivitis, periodontal diseases. Effective against anaerobic microbes.

Main side effects: Nausea, diarrhoea, bad taste, peripheral neuropathies (especially in patients with liver disease).

Contraindications: Pregnancy.

Interactions: Warfarin (increases its effects), alcohol (disulfiram-type reactions).

Adult dose: 200-400 mg, 8-hourly (take with meals).

Minocycline

Class: Tetracycline.

Indications: Mucous membrane pemphigoid. Used for its anti-inflammatory activity.

Main side effects: It can cause vertigo, oral and skin pigmentation.

Contraindications: Pregnancy and children.

Interactions: Not known.

Adult dose: 100-200 mg/daily.

Vancomycin

Class: Glycopeptide.

Indications: Oral bacterial infections in patients allergic to penicillin.

Main side effects: Nausea, fever, phlebitis, rashes, hearing loss, nephrotoxicity.

Contraindications: Renal or auditory impairment.

Interactions: None.

Adult dose: 500 mg, 4 times/daily (orally or intravenously) or 1g, 2 times/daily intravenously.

Antifungal Agents
(for oral candidosis)

Amphotericin (topical)

Indications: Mild candidosis.

Main side effects: None.

Contraindications: None.

Interactions: None.

Adult dose: 4-5 daily mouth washes (oral suspension 100 mg/mL).

Fluconazole

Indications: Useful against candidosis resistant to standard topical treatments, especially in subjects with immunosuppression.

Main side effects: Abdominal pain, nausea, diarrhoea, hepatic toxicity.

Contraindications: Pregnancy, children with renal disease. Less hepatotoxic than ketoconazole.

Interactions: Same as ketaconazole (below).

Adult dose: 50-100 mg, daily; 2-3 daily mouth washes (suspension).

Itraconazole

Indications: Useful against candidosis resistant to standard treatments.

Main side effects: Nausea, vomiting, headaches, rash, oedema.

Contraindications: Pregnancy and breastfeeding.

Interactions: Absorption is reduced by antacids; it increases the effects of ciclosporin, hypoglycaemic agents, diciumarol, digitalis and antihistamines.

Adult dose: Each tablet contains 200-400 mg, daily.

Ketoconazole

Indications: Useful against candidosis resistant to standard treatments.

Main side effects: Nausea, hepatic toxicity.

Contraindications: Pregnancy, patients with chronic hepatic disease.

Interactions: Cimetidine and ranitidine (absorption reduced), isoniazid and rifampicin (effect reduced), antidiabetic drugs (increase the effects). It increases the nephrotoxicity of ciclosporin.

Adult dose: 200-400 mg, daily.

Nystatin

Indications: Candidosis in immunocompetent subjects.

Main side effects: Unpleasant taste, nausea, gastric conditions.

Contraindications: None.

Interactions: None.

Adult dose: 4-6 daily mouth washes (oral suspension 100000 units per mL).

Miconazole (topical)

Indications: Candidosis in immunocompetent subjects. In theory, better antifungal for the treatment of angular cheilitis.

Main side effects: Nausea.

Contraindications: None.

Interactions: None.

Adult dose: 3-4 daily applications of 5 mL gel (25 mg/mL).

Antiviral Agents
(oral herpetic infections)

Aciclovir

Indications: Primary and recurrent herpes simplex virus infection (HSV), and varicella-zoster virus infection (VZV).

Main side effects: Headaches, gastric conditions, rash.

Contraindications: Pregnancy.

Interactions: It increases the renal toxicity of gentamicin, vancomycin, amphotericin and ciclosporin, zidovudine, interferon, alcohol and cocaine (neurological changes).

Adult dose: 5 tablets daily (of 200-400 mg, one every 4 hours) until the primary HSV infection has cleared, for recurrent labial infections and intraoral and for varicella; 800 mg, 5 tablets daily for the zoster. Cream (5%): 4-6 daily applications for recurrent labial lesions. 250 mg/m^2 IV every 8 hours for immunocompromised patients.

Foscarnet

Indications: Aciclovir-resistant HSV or VZV.

Main side effects: Nephrotoxicity, nausea, vomiting, anaemia, fatigue.

Contraindications: Renal disorders.

Interactions: Renal toxicity increases with amphotericin B, pentamidine and aminoglycosides; pentamidine increases the risk of hypocalcaemia.

Adult dose: 40 mg/kg, daily intravenous every 8 hours.

Penciclovir

Indications: Primary and recurrent herpes simplex virus infection (HSV).

Main side effects: None.

Contraindications: None.

Interactions: None.

Adult dose: Cream 1%; 1 application every 2 hours/daily (during the day).

Valaciclovir

Indications: Varicella-zoster infections.

Main side effects: Nausea, headaches, vomiting.

Contraindications: Immunocompromised patients.

Interactions: Cimetidine and probenecid reduce haematological problems.

Adult dose: 1g, 3 times daily.

Corticosteroids

Topical corticosteroids

The European Classification System has four levels numbered I to IV in descending order of potency to classify the clinical potency of corticosteroids: very potent (class I), potent (II), moderately potent (III) and midly potent (IV). Class I and II of topical steroids are usually preferred for the oral cavity, especially in the treatment of erosive bullous diseases. In the case of minor aphthae, a less potent cortisoid might be used. The greatest problem when using topical corticosteroids in the oral cavity is to make adherence to the mucosa possible for as long as it is necessary in order to carry out the treatment. For this, adhesive gels are used, which have a base of carboximethylcellulose (for instance, Orabase[1]) or hydroxyethylcellulose (to 4%) that are mixed in equal parts (50:50) with the topical steroid.

They are often used as an ointment because creams have a bitter taste and the gels can burn because they usually contain alcohol. In any case, it is possible to use salves that provide the paste with greater consistency but less adherence. In the case of gingival lesions, it is often useful to use a tray prepared in transparent soft resin or silicone

---

[1] Not on market release in Italy any longer.

that allows occlusive therapy. The most frequent side effect during a course of topical steroid treatment is candidosis, which is easily prevented with the help of antifungal treatments in the form of chlorhexidine mouthwash and miconazole gel.

Triamcinolone acetonide

Indications: Moderately potent (III).

Main side effects: Oral candidosis.

Contraindications: None.

Interactions: None.

Adult dose: 3-6 daily applications.

Fluocinonide

Indications: Erosive-bullous diseases. Used with adhesive gels of carboximethylcellulose (Orabase); potent (II).

Main side effects: Oral candidosis.

Contraindications: None.

Interactions: None.

Adult dose: 3-6 daily applications.

Clobetasol propionate

Indications: Erosive-bullous diseases. Used with adhesive gels of carboximethylcellulose (Orabase); very potent (class I).

Main side effects: Oral candidosis. Very rarely adrenocortical suppression.

Contraindications: None.

Interactions: None.

Adult dose: 2-3 daily applications.

Systemic corticosteroids

Prednisone

Indications: Severe erosive-bullous diseases (pemphigus mucous membrane pemphigoid, erythema multiforme, and sometimes erosive lichen planus and major aphthae or herpetiform ones).

Main side effects: Gastric irritation, mood swings, insomnia, water retention, hyperglycaemia, weight gain, arterial hypertension, osteoporosis, adrenocortical abolition (Cushingoid aspect).

Contraindications: Pregnancy, osteoporosis, decompensated diabetes, peptic ulcer, hepatic diseases, and psychosis.

Interactions: Anticoagulants and oral antidiabetics (they reduce the effects), NSAIDs (increases the risk of peptic ulcer), furosemide (hypopotassaemia).

Adult dose: 0.5-25 mg/kg orally, once/daily.

Other Immunomodulant Drugs

Azathioprine

Indications: Severe erosive-bullous diseases (pemphigus or mucous membrane pemphigoid). Together with corticosteroids in order to improve their immunosuppressant effectiveness.

Main side effects: Myelosuppression and hepatic toxicity. Chronic use might make the subject susceptible to malignant tumours.

Contraindications: Pregnancy.

Interaction: Allopurinol (it increases azathioprine action), acetylsalicylic acid (bleeding), other immunosuppressants (increased risk of infections).

Adult dose: 2-2.5 mg/kg orally.

Ciclosporin (topical)

Indications: Severe erosive-bullous diseases (pemphigus, mucous membrane pemphigoid, and erosive lichen planus). It can be used as a mouthwash or adhesive base similar to Orabase.

Main side effects: Renal and hepatic toxicity, hypertension, and gingival hyperplasia. All these side effects are rare when the drug is used topically.

Interactions: Allopurinol, analgesics and antifungals (increase toxicity of ciclosporin), antiepileptic drugs (reduction of effects)

Adult dose: 1-10 mouth washes, daily (oral suspension 100 mg/mL); 1-2 daily applications in adhesive base similar to Orabase.

Dapsone

Indications: Mucous membrane pemphigoid.

Main side effects: Anaemia, rash, neuropathy, headaches, renal and hepatic toxicity.

Contraindications: Deficit of glucose-6-phosphate dehydrogenase, pregnancy, and cardiorespiratory diseases.

Interactions: Trimethoprim and methotrexate increase the risk of haematological complications.

Adult dose: 5 mg, daily for the first three days, then 10 mg, daily for the next three days, and then 15 mg, daily for the next three days; then 20 mg, daily.

Tacrolimus (topical)

Indications: lichen planus, pemphigoid.

Main side effects: Burning sensation.

Contraindications: None.

Interactions: None.

Adult dose: 1-2 daily applications.

Other Drugs

Carbamazepine

Indications: Trigeminal neuralgia.

Main side effects: Occasional vertigo, diplopia and haematological dyscrasia, usually with rash in the first three months of treatment.

Contraindications: Deficit of glucose-6-phosphate dehydrogenase, pregnancy, and cardiorespiratory diseases.

Interactions: Enhanced by cimetidine and isoniazide, it increases the effect of lithium; it interferes with oral contraceptives.

Adult dose: Usually start with 200 mg, daily. Many patients need 200 mg every 8 hours; do not exceed 1800 mg, daily.

Pilocarpine

Indications: Xerostomia.

Main side effects: Sweating, bradycardia, tachycardia, hypotension-hypertension, and biliary spasm.

Contraindications: Hypertension, cardiovascular diseases, arrhythmia, psychosis, urinary lithiasis and biliary diseases.

Interactions: Betablocker (risk of arrhythmia), anticholinergic (compromises its effects), cholinergic (increases its action).

Adult dose: 1 teaspoon, 1-4 times daily (solution 5 mg/mL).

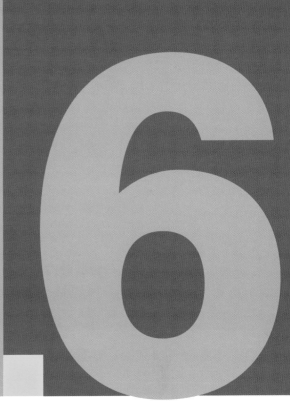

Chapter Six

Main drug side effects of oral and perioral localisation

Most side effects from oral and perioral drugs tend to be rare. This section lists only the most common ones. The identification of the pharmacological agent responsible for the side effects is mostly clinical, by establishing a temporal relation between the introduction of the drug and its clinical manifestation, and also thanks to the bibliographical research of similar cases published in the relevant literature. There are no accurate and/or specific biological tests that can help with the diagnosis. For further information please refer to the pharmacopoeia.

Angioedema

- Acetylsalicylic acid
- Captopril
- Carbamazepine
- Cephalosporins
- Co-trimoxazole
- Iodide contrast media
- Penicillins

Candidosis

- Broad-spectrum antibiotics
- Corticosteroids (topical and systemic)
- Immunosuppressants

Cheilitis

- Cytotoxic drugs
- Lithium
- Penicillamine
- Retinoids

Erythema Multiforme

- Allopurinol[1]
- Barbiturates*
- Carbamazepine
- Cephalosporins
- Co-trimoxazole*
- Phenylbutazone*
- Phenytoin
- Phenolphthalein
- Phenothiazines
- Hydantoin
- Oxyphenylbutazone

- Penicillins*
- Piroxicam*
- Pyrazolones*
- Sulfonamides

Pain in Salivary Glands

- Guanethidine

Gingival Swelling

- Ciclosporin
- Phenytoin
- Nifedipine (and other calcium channel blockers)

Hypersalivation

- Anticholinesterases

Lichenoid Reactions

- Antimalarials
- Non-steroidal anti-inflammatory drugs (NSAID).
- Beta blockers
- Captopril
- Phenytoin
- Methyldopa
- Para-aminosalicylate
- Penicillamine
- Procainamide
- Sulphonamides

Black Hairy Tongue

- Iron salts
- Griseofulvin

Lupoid Reactions
(lupus-like)

- Hydralazine
- Procainamide

Oral Pigmentation

- Chloroquine
- Mepacrine

---

[1] * Drugs that more frequently cause severe forms of erythema multiforme (Stevens-Johnson syndrome and toxic epidermal necrolysis)

Osteochemonecrosis

- Bisphosphonates

Pemphigus Vulgaris

- Penicillamine
- Rifampicin

Pemphigoid-Like Reactions

- Clonidine
- Psoralens

Dental Pigmentation

- Chlorhexidine
- Iron
- Tetracylines[2]

Trigeminal Paraesthesia

- Acetazolamide
- Labetalol
- Sulthiame

Xerostomia

- Alfuzosin
- Amoxapine
- Tricyclic antidepressants

[2] Minocycline can cause dental pigmentation in adults, whilst tetracycline can stain the teeth in the course of their development.

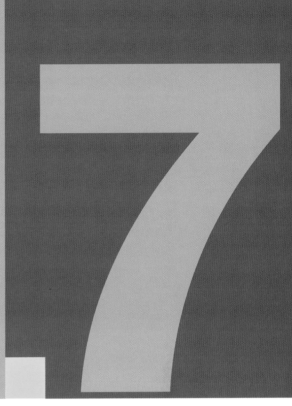

Chapter Seven

Therapeutic protocols

Herpetic Infection

Herpes simplex

1. Primary herpetic gingivostomatitis:
Aciclovir, 1g, daily until lesions clear. It is also helpful to follow a light diet with adequate hydration; antipyretics/analgesics (paracetamol/ acetoaminophen); local antiseptics (rinse with chlorhexidine).

2. Labial and intraoral recurrent herpes:
Penciclovir cream, 6 daily applications (seems to be more effective than aciclovir against labial herpes). In immunocompromised people, aciclovir, 1-2 g, daily until the lesions clear (the dosage depends on the seriousness of the clinical manifestations and on the immune status).

Herpes zoster

Valaciclovir, 3 g, daily for 7 days, or famciclovir, 500 mg, daily for 7 days, or aciclovir, 4 g, daily for 7-10 days. Valaciclovir is the drug of first choice. In the case of immunocompromised patients who are aciclovir-resistant, foscarnet, 40 mg/kg intravenous every 8 hours for 10 days. Prednisone 60 mg, daily for 7 days, 30 mg may help, daily for 7 days, and 15 mg, daily for 7 days to relieve pain and oedema in the acute phase, but it does not reduce the incidence of post-herpetic neuralgia.

Oral Candidosis

1. Angular cheilitis in immunocompetent patients:
Miconazole oral gel, 3 applications daily.

2. Prosthesis-induced candidosis:
Miconazole oral gel, 3 applications daily. Treat the removable prosthesis by applying conditioners and soaking the prosthesis in a solution of hypochlorite or nystatin (at least for 1 hour per day).

3. Erythematous or pseudomembranous candidosis in immunocompetent patients:
Topical therapy: chlorhexidine in water solution, 3 daily mouthwashes plus miconazole oral gel (or fluconazole in suspension), 3 daily applications.

Systemic therapy: (including angular cheilitis).

4. Hyperplastic candidosis in immunocompetent patients:
Topical therapy: as in 3 above, plus surgery. Fluconazole, 50 mg, daily for 14 days, or 10 mg for 3 days and 50 mg for the following 8 days.

5. Erythematous or pseudomembranous candidosis or angular cheilitis in immunocompromised patients:
Fluconazole, 50 mg, daily for 14 days, or 100 mg for 3 days and 50 mg for the following 8 days.

In case of fluconazole-resistant strains: Itraconazole 200-400 mg, daily; in case of resistance to itraconazole use ketoconazole, 200 mg, daily for 3-5 weeks.

Algorithm for the Treatment of Oral Candidosis

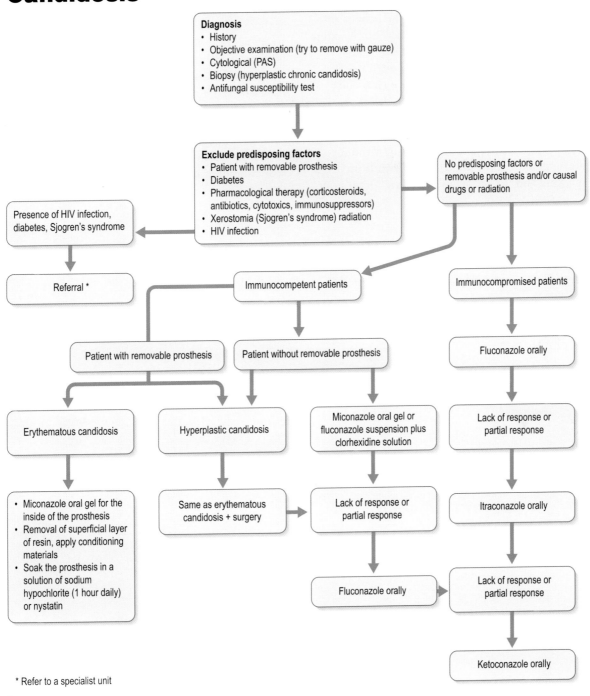

* Refer to a specialist unit

FIGURE 7.1 Algorithm for treatment of oral candidosis.

Recurrent Aphthous Stomatitis

Exclude possible associated diseases.

1. Minor aphthae: Reassure the patient and only initiate treatment if requested. Chlorhexidine solution or gel, 3 times daily ; if there is no response or only a partial response then use triamcinolone acetonide in adhesive (3-6 daily applications), or fluocinonide (3-6, daily) or clobetasol ointment (2, daily) until ulcers clear. Before applying topical corticosteroids, dry the area in question then apply the drug without pressing and ask the patient to abstain from speaking and/or eating and drinking for an hour.

2. Major aphthae: Fluocinonide or clobetasol ointment in adhesive gel (2-3 daily applications). If the treatment lasts any longer than a week, add an antimycotic agent such as chlorhexidine solution (3 days) plus miconazole oral gel (1 day). If there is no response or if lesions are not treatable topically due to their location, then use prednisone 50 mg, daily until there is a reduction of at least 50% of the lesions and then decrease dose slowly.

3. Herpetiform aphthae: Prednisone 50 mg, daily for 3 days, 25 mg, daily for 3 days, then 3 tablets every other day until there is a reduction of at least 50% of the lesions.

Algorithm for the Treatment of Recurrent Aphthous Stomatitis

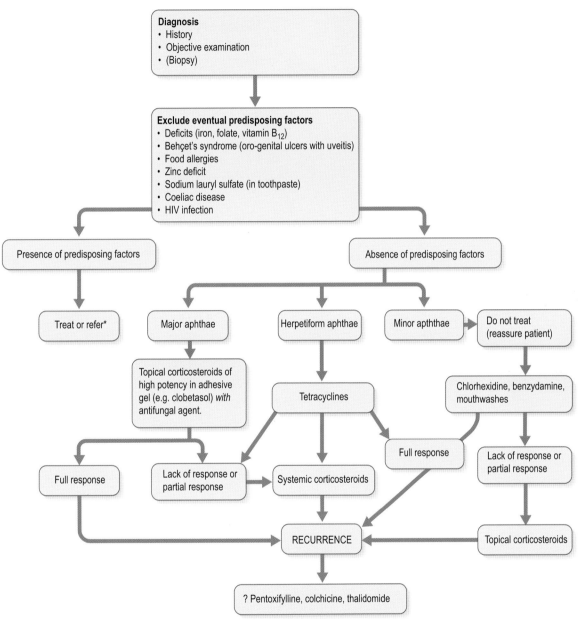

* Refer to a specialist unit

FIGURE 7.2 Algorithm for treatment of recurrent aphthous stomatitis.

Erythema Multiforme

1. Oral erythema multiforme: Stop any potential triggering drug. Clobetasol ointment in adhesive gel (2 daily) with antifungal prophylaxis until it improves by 50%, then 1 daily until the lesion clears completely. Before applying topical corticosteroids, dry the area in question then apply the drug and ask the patient to abstain from speaking and/or eating and drinking for an hour. In case of widespread oral lesions or lesions not amenable to topical treatment, use prednisone 50 mg, daily for 3 days, 25 mg, daily for 3 days, and then 3 tablets every other day.

2. Minor erythema multiforme: If related to HSV, aciclovir (1-2 g, daily) until the lesions improve by 50%, then decrease. If not related to HSV, oral lesions to be treated as in 1. Cutaneous lesions, hydroxyzine (50 mg, daily) and topical steroids if required.

3. Major erythema multiforme (Stevens-Johnson's syndrome): If medication-induced, discontinue the drugs and use prednisone, 50 mg, daily for 3 days; 25 mg, daily for 3 days, then 25 mg every other day until there is a 50% healing of the lesions. Then decrease the dosage slowly. If the cause is *Mycoplasma pneumoniae* then use erythromycin (0.5-1 g, daily).

Algorithm for the Treatment of Erythema Multiforme

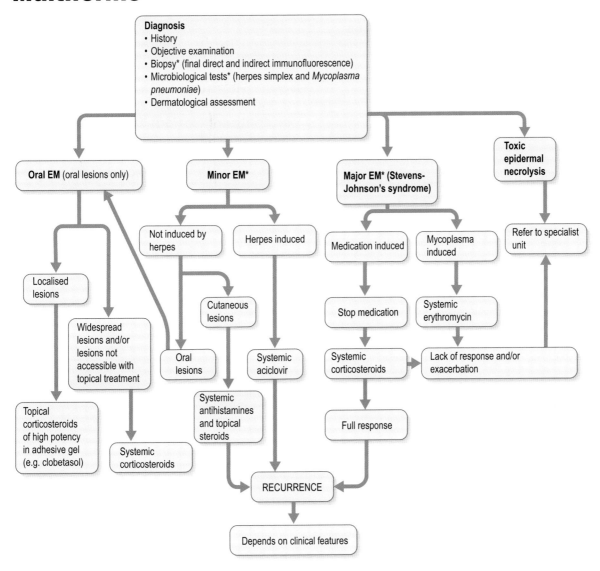

Diagnosis
- History
- Objective examination
- Biopsy* (final direct and indirect immunofluorescence)
- Microbiological tests* (herpes simplex and *Mycoplasma pneumoniae*)
- Dermatological assessment

Oral EM (oral lesions only)

Minor EM*

Major EM* (Stevens-Johnson's syndrome)

Toxic epidermal necrolysis

Localised lesions

Widespread lesions and/or lesions not accessible with topical treatment

Not induced by herpes

Herpes induced

Medication induced

Mycoplasma induced

Refer to specialist unit

Cutaneous lesions

Stop medication

Systemic erythromycin

Topical corticosteroids of high potency in adhesive gel (e.g. clobetasol)

Oral lesions

Systemic aciclovir

Systemic corticosteroids

Lack of response and/or exacerbation

Systemic corticosteroids

Systemic antihistamines and topical steroids

Full response

RECURRENCE

Depends on clinical features

* Refer to a specialist unit

FIGURE 7.3 Algorithm for treatment of erythema multiforme (EM).

Lichen Planus

Begin by treating symptomatic areas (usually atrophic-erosive), after having considered the elimination of potential predisposing factors.

1. Exclusively oral clinical features amenable to topical treatment:

Clobetasol ointment in adhesive gel (twice daily) for 2 months, then once daily for another month with antifungal prophylaxis (chlorhexidine plus miconazole). Before applying the topical corticosteroid, dry the area in question then apply the drug without pressing and ask the patient to abstain from speaking and/or eating and drinking for an hour. If lesions are gingival, prepare trays for occlusive therapy.

2. Exclusively oral clinical features not amenable to topical treatment or mucous-cutaneous features:

Prednisone 50 mg, daily for 3 days, 25 mg, daily for 3 days, then 25 mg every other day until an improvement of 50% of the lesion and then decrease the dosage slowly. If necessary combine azathioprine (50 mg, daily). Maintenance with topical treatment as in 1 above.

3. Lack of response to corticosteroids or contraindications for their use:

Tacrolimus 0.03% ointment (twice daily).

Algorithm for the Treatment of Lichen Planus

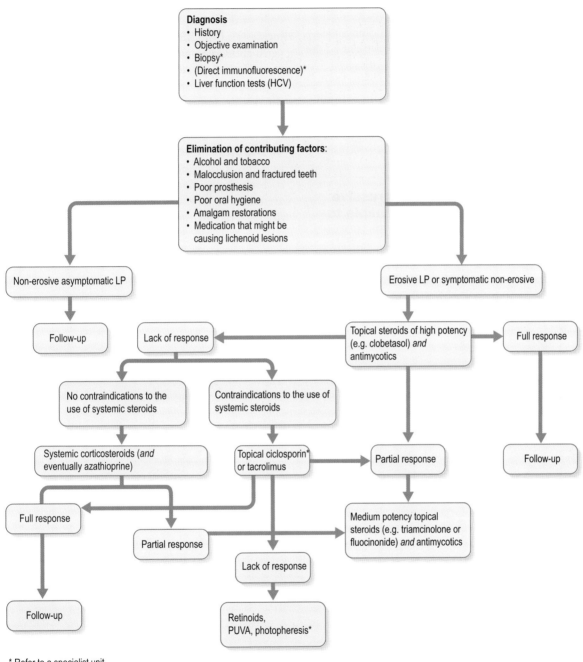

* Refer to a specialist unit

FIGURE 7.4 Algorithm for treatment of lichen planus (LP).

Mucous Membrane Pemphigoid

1. Exclusively oral clinical features that are amenable to topical treatment:

Clobetasol ointment in adhesive gel (twice daily), with antifungal prophylaxis (chlorhexidine plus miconazole) until at least 75% improvement of the lesions, and then slowly decrease the dosage. Before applying the topical corticosteroids, dry the area in question then apply the drug without pressing and ask the patient to abstain from speaking and/or eating and drinking for an hour. If lesions are gingival, prepare trays for occlusive therapy.

2. Lack of response, or progressive disease, or disease not amenable to topical treatment:

Prednisone 50-100 mg, daily (according to the severity of the clinical features) until there is at least a 50% improvement of the lesions, and then decrease the dosage slowly and combine it with the topical treatment described in 1 above.

3. Lack of response, or progressive disease, or disease not amenable to topical treatment *(oral cavity only)* and contraindications to the use of systemic steroids:

Minocycline 100 mg, daily or dapsone, 25 mg for the first 3 days, then increasing from 25 mg every 3 days to 150 mg (give cimetidine and vitamin E to minimise haemolysis. In both cases the aim is to obtain an improvement of at least 50% and then to decrease the dosage and to combine with the topical treatment described in 1 above.

4. Disease involving other mucosae:

As in 2 above, or azathioprine (1-2 mg/kg) daily or cyclophosphamide (0.5-2 mg/kg, daily) if there are ocular lesions, or dapsone (see 3 above for the dosage), or sulfapyridine (1.5-3 g, daily).

Algorithm for the Treatment of Mucous Membrane Pemphigoid

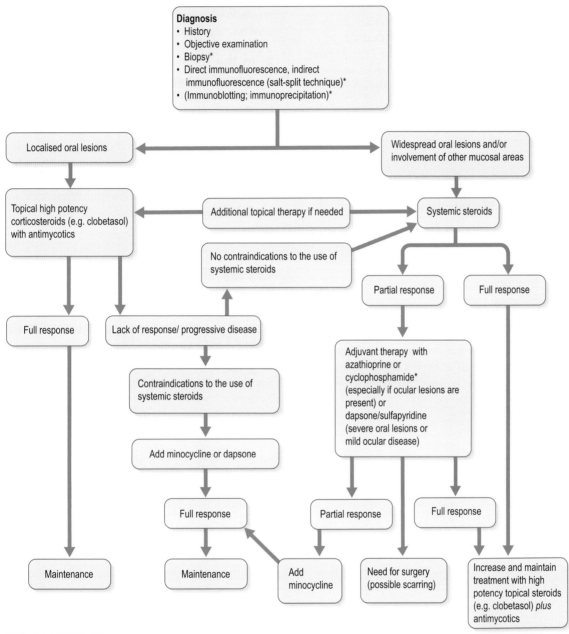

Diagnosis
- History
- Objective examination
- Biopsy*
- Direct immunofluorescence, indirect immunofluorescence (salt-split technique)*
- (Immunoblotting; immunoprecipitation)*

Localised oral lesions

Widespread oral lesions and/or involvement of other mucosal areas

Topical high potency corticosteroids (e.g. clobetasol) with antimycotics

Additional topical therapy if needed

Systemic steroids

No contraindications to the use of systemic steroids

Full response

Lack of response/ progressive disease

Partial response

Full response

Adjuvant therapy with azathioprine or cyclophosphamide* (especially if ocular lesions are present) or dapsone/sulfapyridine (severe oral lesions or mild ocular disease)

Contraindications to the use of systemic steroids

Add minocycline or dapsone

Full response

Partial response

Full response

Maintenance

Maintenance

Add minocycline

Need for surgery (possible scarring)

Increase and maintain treatment with high potency topical steroids (e.g. clobetasol) *plus* antimycotics

* Refer to a specialist unit

FIGURE 7.5 Algorithm for treatment of mucous membrane pemphigoid.

Pemphigus Vulgaris

Pemphigus vulgaris is a disease that can be potentially fatal. For this reason, treatment must be given not just according to the clinical features and the immunological data (antiepithelial antibody titres from indirect immunofluorescence or ELISA), but also to possible associated conditions (see Mucous Membrane Pemphigoid, above), where a systemic corticosteroid in high dosage and for a prolonged period might be contraindicated or where the lesions determine the need for adjuvant treatment. This section offers general treatment recommendations. It is important to monitor the patient periodically in terms of blood pressure, haematological profile, electrolytes, blood sugar levels, bone density and the possibility of intercurrent infections.

1. Exclusively oral clinical features amenable to topical treatment:

Clobetasol ointment in adhesive gel (2, daily), with antifungal prophylaxis (chlorhexidine plus miconazole) until the lesions have improved by at least 75%, and then slowly decrease the dosage. Before applying topical corticosteroids, dry the area in question then apply the drug without pressing and ask the patient to abstain from speaking and/or eating and drinking for an hour. If lesions are gingival, prepare trays for occlusive therapy. If there is only a partial response or no response at all to the treatment, add dapsone (see Mucous Membrane Pemphigoid above) or systemic tetracycline or move onto treatment with systemic steroids.

2. In the case of widespread oral involvement and/or involvement of more mucosal or cutaneous areas:

Prednisone 50-100 mg, daily, plus azathioprine (1-2 mg/kg) daily, or cyclophosphamide (0.5-2 mg/kg, daily) (based on the seriousness of the clinical features). Once positive results have been obtained, increase the steroid slowly and maintain with the second immunosuppressor and topical steroids. Mycophenolate mofetil or ciclosporin are alternatives.

Oral Keratosis

See the relevant algorithm.

Burning Mouth Syndrome

See the relevant algorithm.

Algorithm for the Treatment of Pemphigus Vulgaris

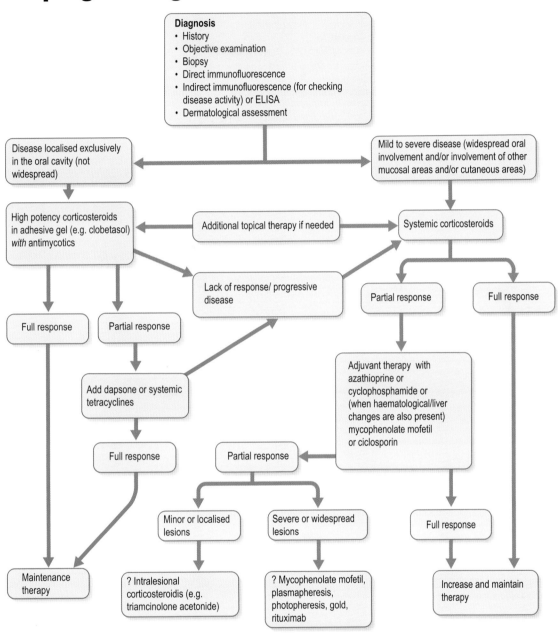

FIGURE 7.6 Algorithm for treatment of pemphigus vulgaris.

Algorithm for Oral Keratosis

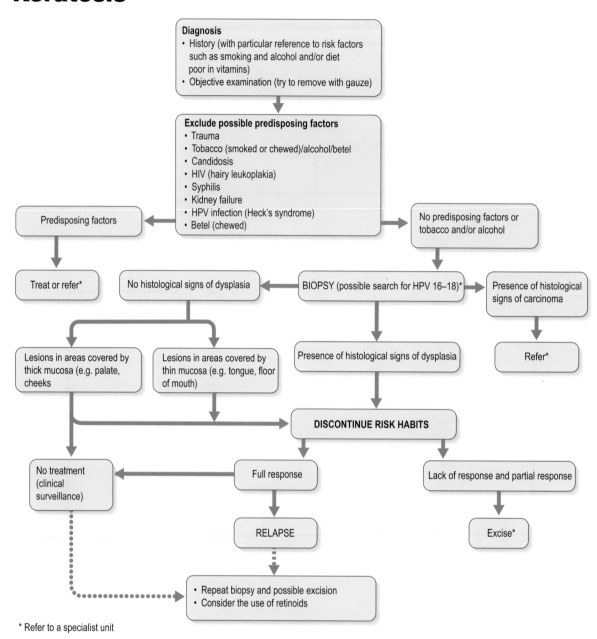

FIGURE 7.7 Algorithm for treatment of oral keratosis.

Algorithm for Burning Mouth Syndrome

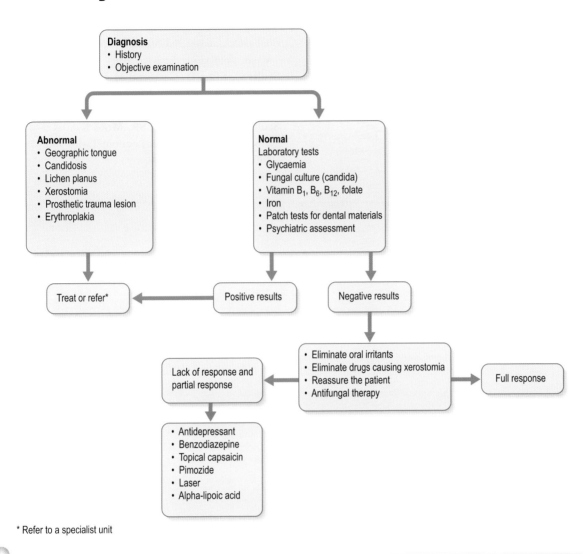

* Refer to a specialist unit

FIGURE 7.8 Algorithm for treatment of burning mouth syndrome.

References

AAVV Third European Congress of Oral Medicine. Oral Dis 1997; 3:43-48

Carbone M, Conrotto D, Carrozzo M, Broccoletti R, Gandolfo S, Scully C Topical corticorallyteroids in association with miconazole and chlorhexidine in the long-term management of atrophic-erorallyive oral lichen planus: a placebo-controlled and comparative study between clobetasol and fluocinonide. Oral Dis 1999; 5:44-49

Huang W, Rothe MJ, Grant-Kels JM The burning mouth syndrome. J Am Acad Dermatol 1996; 34:91-98

Katsambas AD, Lotti TM European handbook of dermatological treatment. Berlin: Springer-Verlag, 1999

Scully C, Carrozzo M, Gandolfo S, Puiatti P, Monteil R Update on mucous membrane pemphigoid, a heterogeneous immue-mediated sub-epithelial blistering entity. Oral Surg Oral Med Oral Pathol Oral Radiol End 1999; 88:56-68

Scully C, Cawson RA Medical problems in dentistry, 5th ed. Edinburgh: Elsevier, 2004

Scully C, Eisen D, Carrozzo M The management of oral lichen planus. Am J Clin Dermatol 2000; 1(5): 287-306

Scully C, Flint S, Porter SR, Moos K Atlas of oral and maxillofacial disease. London: Taylor and Martin, 2004

Part Four

Biopsies and vital stains

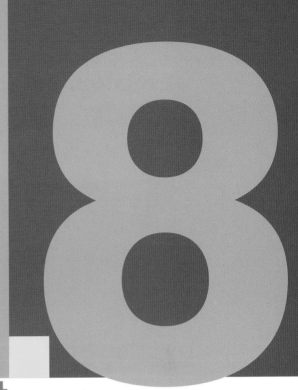

Chapter Eight

How to perform a biopsy of the oral mucosa

First, you must decide what type of biopsy is required, excisional or incisional.

Excisional Biopsy

Excisional biopsies are reserved for superficial lesions no larger than 1cm maximum.

Warning

If a malignant tumour is suspected, however small, excisional biopsy must be carried out by a specialist. Due to the dangerous nature of the procedure (both in terms of diagnosis and therapy), the patient's life could be at risk if mistakes are made.

If you are not an expert, refer the patient to a specialist.

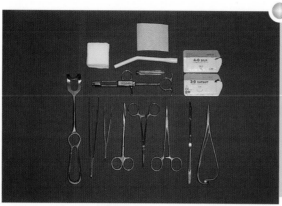

FIGURE 8.1 Instruments for excisional biopsy:
Middeldorpf hook
Suction tube
Scalpel blade no. 15
Surgical pliers
Anatomical clamp
Scissors
Suture threads (catgut or silk of 000 or 0000)
2 Klemmer forceps
Needle holder
Cartridge-type anaesthetic syringe
Paper.

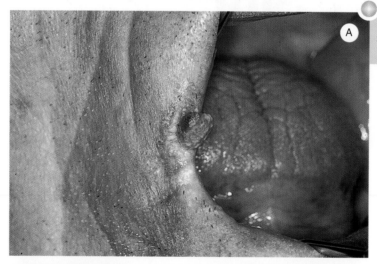

A

FIGURE 8.2 An excisional biopsy must be reserved for superficial lesions no larger than 1 cm maximum.

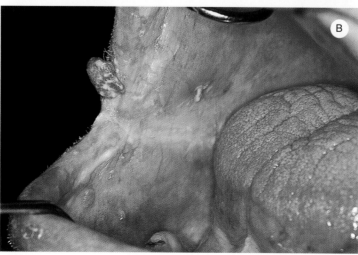

B

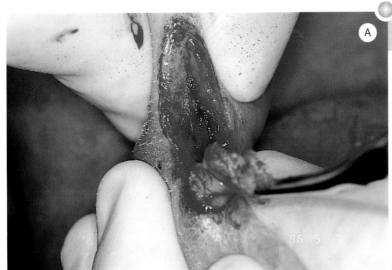

FIGURE 8.3 The excision must be complete, even in case of carcinoma.

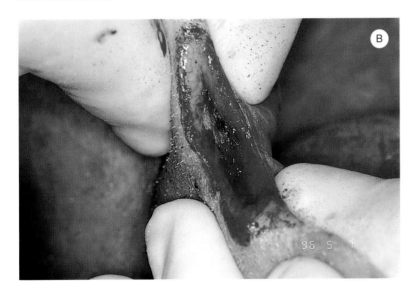

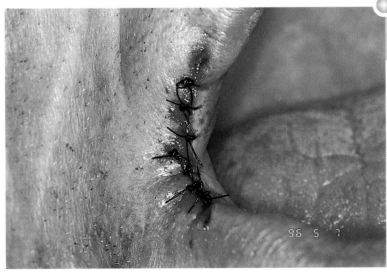

FIGURE 8.4 Finally, after having performed haemostasis, closure is by suture.

Incisional Biopsy

Incisional biopsy consists of taking one or more significant samples from the lesion for diagnosis.

Choosing the area where the biopsy is best carried out is based on two possibilities:

- assessment of the clinical appearance
- vital toluidine blue staining.

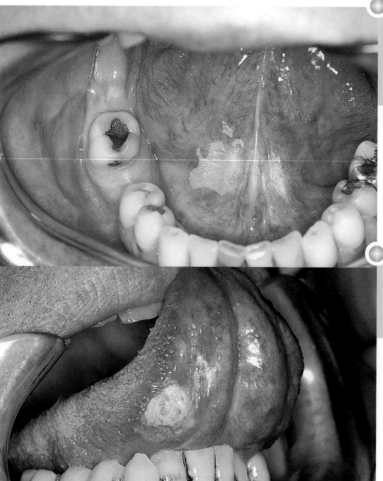

FIGURE 8.5 A **simple incisional biopsy** consists of taking a sample with representative healthy and diseased tissue from the lesion. This is indicated for homogeneous lesions, usually white spots or plaques.

FIGURE 8.6 A **simple incisional biopsy** can be performed also in non-homogeneous lesions, taking the sample from the most suspicious area (generally red areas or areas with erosions).

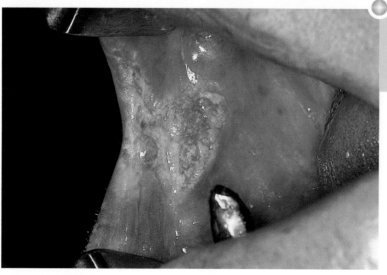

FIGURE 8.7 A **mapping incisional biopsy** consists of taking more samples, each from a clinically significant area for diagnosis. This is usually performed on non-homogeneous lesions.

Steps to follow for an incisional biopsy

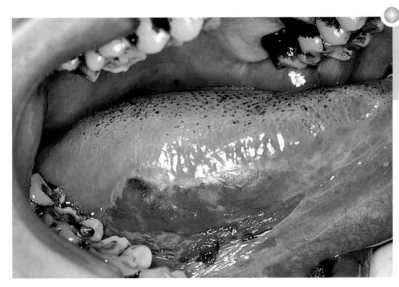

FIGURE 8.8 The **guided incisional biopsy** is preceded by vital staining with **toluidine blue** (see Chapter 9). This is performed on non-homogeneous lesions with predominant red areas.

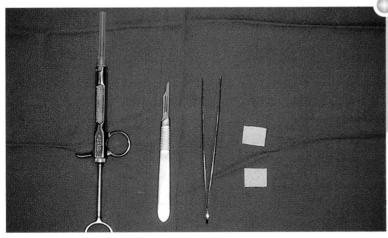

FIGURE 8.9 Step 1 Instruments.
Instruments for incisional biopsy:
Scalpel blade no. 15
Surgical pliers
Cartridge-type anaesthetic syringe
Paper
Those instruments needed for suture must be ready but only if necessary.

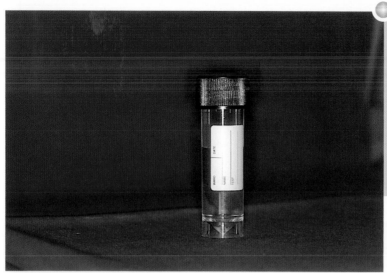

FIGURE 8.10 Step 2 Fixing solution (fixative).
The most commonly used is the 10% formalin. Prepare a container that:
Is large enough because the volume of formalin is three times the specimen to be taken
Has a watertight top
Has a self-adhesive label to write the name of the patient on immediately after the sample is taken (and date, time and unit number).

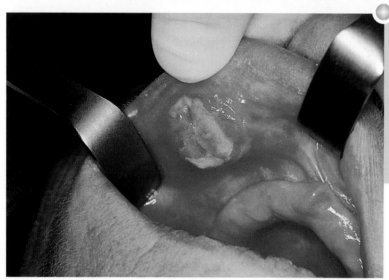

FIGURE 8.11 Step 3 Preliminary considerations. Before performing the biopsy, assess the lesion carefully and decide the following:
What type of incisional biopsy is required?
Which area the samples must be taken from?
How useful is it to use the toluidine blue staining?
The choice is essentially based on the clinical appearance of the lesion in question.

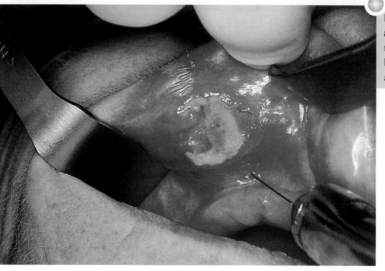

FIGURE 8.12 Step 4. Local anaesthetic. Do not inject directly into the lesion and do not apply pressure because the tissues might be damaged and artefacts might be introduced.

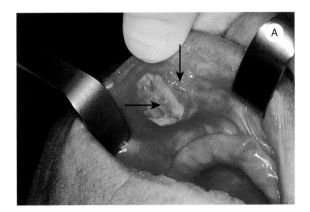

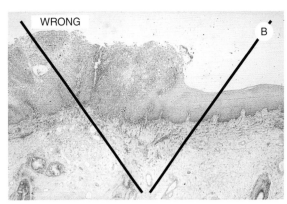

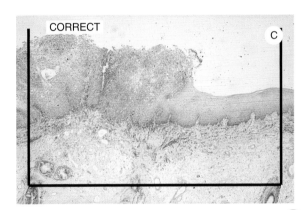

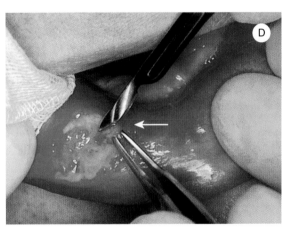

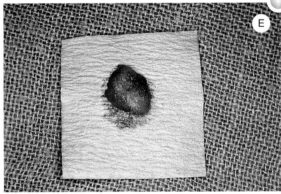

FIGURE 8.13 Step 5. Taking the samples.

Never sample an area of necrosis (A).

Include also some healthy tissue (A).

The incision must not be wedge-shaped since it includes a small amount of lamina propria and basal layer (B).

It must be sufficiently deep to allow study of the interface epithelium-connective; this means a pre-operative examination of the depth of the lesion in question (C).

It must be large enough for correct interpretation (at least 4/5 mm).

When using surgical pliers pay attention not to crush or tear the tissues; for the more delicate sampling (e.g. bullous diseases) use anatomical pliers (D).

Put the sample on the paper with the epithelium facing up, which will give better orientation (E).

The sample is immediately fixed with formalin.

Steps to follow for and incisional biopsy preceded by vital staining

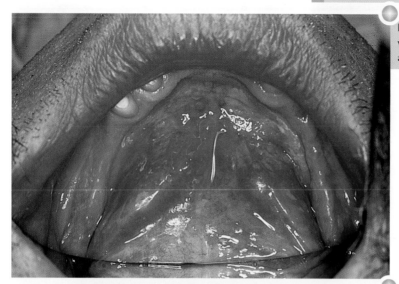

FIGURE 8.14 Vital staining is used when lesions are non-homogeneous, red and white or predominantly red.

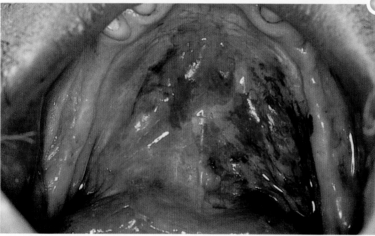

FIGURE 8.15 After performing the staining (see Chapter 9) assess which areas samples need to be taken from, and only select those where the staining is royal blue stain.

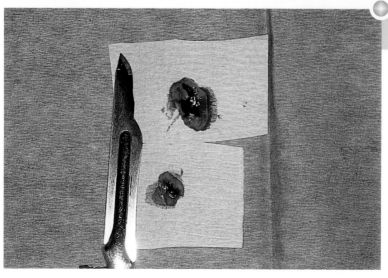

FIGURE 8.16 The sample must also contain areas that have not been stained.

Oral Lichen Planus Biopsy

Whatever the clinical aspect of the lesion in question, the choice for the area where the biopsy will take place follows some guidelines. If possible, the sample must contain one or more **papules** or, alternatively, part of a striated or **plaque-like** lesion. The ideal site is the buccal mucosa.

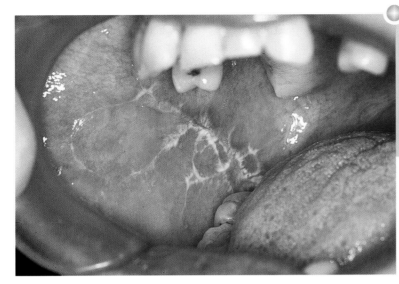

FIGURE 8.17 The surface of the sample must be wide enough (7-8 mm^2) and not too deep. Avoid white plaques on the dorsum of the tongue as much as possible and atrophic red spots because they can be of uncertain histological interpretation. Avoid erosions and ulcers because samples from such sites can be difficult to interpret.

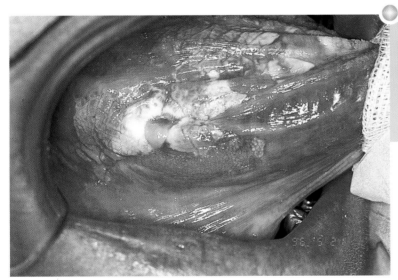

FIGURE 8.18 Remember that **lichen planus** can be a precancerous condition, therefore examine and evaluate carefully the clinical aspects that you wish to subject to biopsy. If there are also lesions that might suggest the presence of early oral cancer, proceed with caution and refer to a specialist unit.

Note

In cases of uncertain diagnosis, it might be useful to carry out direct immunofluorescence that will display linear deposits of fibrin at the basement membrane zone.

Direct immunofluorescence

For suspected autoimmune diseases of the oral mucosa this analysis is essential to clarify the diagnosis. Direct Immunofluorescence Staining (DIF) is carried out by taking a sample of the lesion following the same criteria as for an incisional biopsy. A larger amount of tissue must be provided since a part of it has to be preserved in OCT or in PBS and therefore processed for DIF; the other part is processed via a traditional histology. For possible lichen or lupus, the criteria to follow are those in the previous paragraph. For suspected bullous disease the sample:

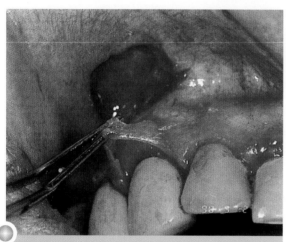

FIGURE 8.19 Sampling carried out in proximity of desquamative gingivitis, avoiding the area in which the epithelium is easily detachable.

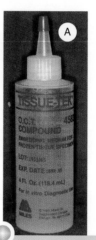
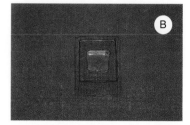

FIGURE 8.20 OCT must be poured out in its container without creating bubbles; the sample must be carefully placed down with the epithelium facing up.

Note

A part of the sample is kept in one of these two ways and immediately taken to a laboratory.

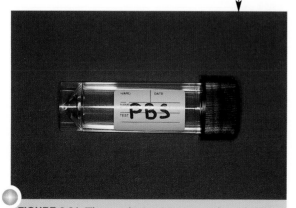

FIGURE 8.21 The sample goes into a test-tube with PBS.

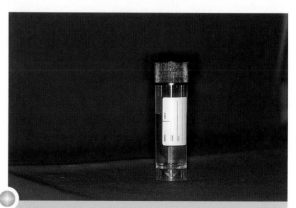

FIGURE 8.22 A part of the sample is fixed in formalin in order to perform a traditional histological evaluation.

- must be carried out in areas where epithelium is present (not erosions)
- all precautions must be taken to avoid tearing the epithelium-connective interface whilst taking the specimen
- it is advised that a sample is taken from the edge of the lesions where the mucosa appears to be healthy and to use forceps.

References

Abbey LM, Kaugars GE, Gunsolley JC, et al The effect of clinical information on histopathologic diagnosis of oral epithelial dysplasia. Oral Surg Oral Med Oral Pathol Oral Radiol Endod 1998; 85:74-77

Bramley PA, Smith CJ Oral cancer and precancer: establishing a diagnosis. Br Dent J 1990; 168:103-107

Ficozzo G, McClintock B, Honsen LS Artifacts created during oral biopsy procedures. J Cranio MaxFac Surg 1987; 15:34-37

Gandolfo S, Carbone M, Carrozzo M, et al Biopsy procedures in the diagnosis of oral cancer: incisional or excisional? Clinical Review. Minerva Stomatol 1993; 42:69-75

Silverman S Jr Early diagnosis of oral cancer. Cancer 1988; 62:1796-1799

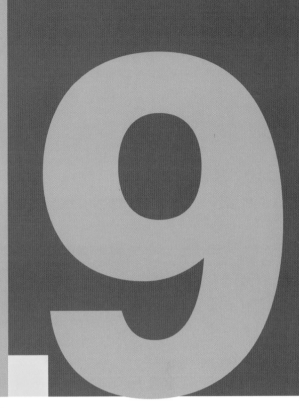

Chapter Nine

How to perform a toluidine blue staining

Note

Box 9.1 Toluidine blue formula (according to Mashberg)

Toluidine blue in powder form	1 g
Acetic acid	10 mL
Pure alcohol	4.19 mL
Distilled water	86 mL

Toluidine blue does not constitute a complete diagnostic technique but it is part of a wider protocol that includes biopsy of toluidine blue positive areas (see *Biopsies* section).

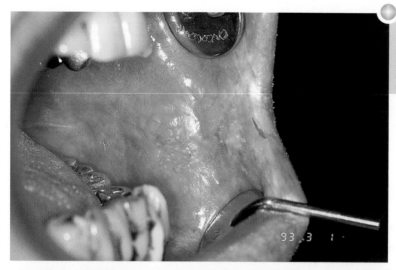

FIGURE 9.1 Careful evaluation of the mucosa allows us to determine lesions that require the use of toluidine blue: red lesions; non-homogeneous white and red lesions; especially if they are multiple and/or extended to one or more areas.

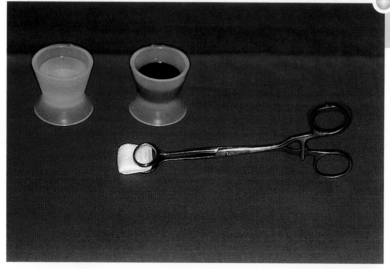

FIGURE 9.2 Necessary equipment: container for acetic acid 1%; container for toluidine blue; ring pliers; gauze.

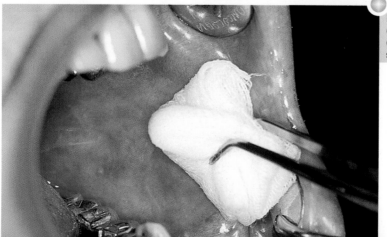

FIGURE 9.3 1. Rinse with water (20 seconds). 2. Rinse with acetic acid 1% (20 seconds). 3. Finally dry the lesional surface.

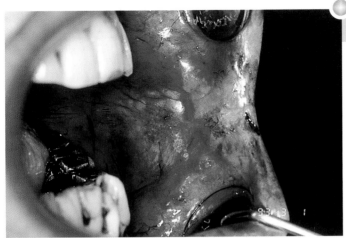

FIGURE 9.4 Apply the stain in excess and leave on site for 1 minute.

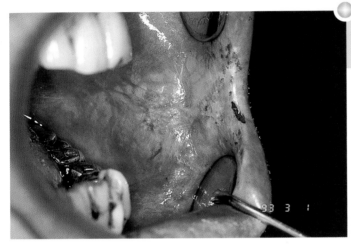

FIGURE 9.5 In order to eliminate excess stain, rinse the lesion again with: 1) acetic acid 1% (20 seconds); 2) sufficient water. **Only the dark blue areas (blue royal) are positive.**

References

Broccoletti R, Carrozzo M, Carbone P, Garzino-Demo P, Gandolfo S A new computer-aided method evaluating toluidine blue staining in oral cancer and precancer. In:.Varma A.K, ed. Oral oncology. Proceeding of the 5th International Congress on oral cancer, September 1997, London, vol. V;124-127.

Epphros H, Mashberg A, Wysocki G, Allen C Toluidine blue – viewpoints. Oral Surg Oral Med Oral Pathol Oral Radiol Endod 1999; 87:526-529

Epstein JB, Scully C, Spinelli JJ Toluidine blue and Lugol's iodine application in the assesment of oral malignant disease and lesions at risk of malignancy. J Oral Patol Med 1992; 21:160-163

Gandolfo S, Pentenezo M, Broccoletti R, et al Toluidine blue uptake in potentially malignant oral lesions in vivo: Clinical and biological assessment. Oral Oncol 2006; 42:89-95

Mashberg A Final evaluation of tolonium chloride rinse for screening of high-risk patients with asymptomatic squamous carcinoma. J Am Dent Assoc 1983; 106:319-323

Mashberg A Tolonium (toluidine blue) rinse a screening method for recognition of squamous cell carcinoma. Cancer 1981; 245:2408-2410

Silverman S Jr, Migliorati C, Bezbosa J Toluidine blue staining in the detection of oral precancerous and malignant lesions. Oral Surg Oral Med Oral Pathol 1984; 54:379-382

Warnakulasuriya KAAS, Johnson NW Sensitivity and specificity of OralScan Toluidine blue mouthrinse in the detection of oral cancer and precancer. J Oral Pathol Med 1996; 25:97-103

Index